Fracture Management Joint by Joint

Series editors

Filippo Castoldi
Department of Orthopaedics
CTO Hospital Turin
Torino
Italy

Davide Edoardo Bonasia
University of Torino
AO Ordine Mauriziano
Torino
Italy

This book series aims to provide orthopedic surgeons with up-to-date practical guidance on the assessment, preoperative work-up, and surgical management of intra-articular fractures involving different joints, including the shoulder, knee, hip, elbow, ankle, and wrist. Complex articular fractures are difficult to treat and sometimes require specific surgical skills appropriate to the involved joint. In addition, arthroscopic-assisted fracture reduction is increasing in popularity, but trauma surgeons are generally not trained in arthroscopic techniques. For these reasons, articular fractures are often referred by the trauma team to surgeons experienced in the management of injuries to the joint in question. Therefore, across the world it is becoming common for orthopedic surgeons to specialize in treating fractures of only one joint. This series is designed to fill a gap in the literature by presenting the shared experience of surgeons skilled in the use of arthroscopic and open techniques on individual joints.

More information about this series at http://www.springer.com/series/13619

Filippo Castoldi
Davide Edoardo Bonasia

Editors

Fractures Around the Knee

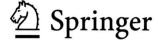 Springer

Editors
Filippo Castoldi
University of Torino
CTO hospital
Torino
Italy

Davide Edoardo Bonasia
University of Torino
AO Ordine Mauriziano
Torino
Italy

Fracture Management Joint by Joint
ISBN 978-3-319-28804-8   ISBN 978-3-319-28806-2   (eBook)
DOI 10.1007/978-3-319-28806-2

Library of Congress Control Number: 2016937325

This Springer imprint is published by Springer Nature
The registered company is Springer International Publishing AG Switzerland

Contents

Stefano Zaffagnini, Federico Raggi,
Alberto Grassi, Tommaso Roberti di Sarsina,
Cecilia Signorelli, and Maurilio Marcacci

Abstract

Patella fractures are relatively rare compared to all skeletal injuries but quite common for those who works with knee trauma. This type of fractures are mainly caused by a direct trauma, and can generally be diagnosed by clinical presentation and x-rays. Conservative treatment is reserved for non-displaced fractures, for other surgical reduction and fixation by tension band tachnique are the best choices.

The surgeon must know postoperative management and how to handle the early and late complications of this type of fractures.

1.1 Epidemiology

Patellar fractures are relatively rare and represent 1 % of all skeletal injuries [1, 2] with an overall incidence of 10.7 per 100.000 people per year [3]. This type of fractures is most common in the age range of 20–50 years, and the incidence in men is almost twice than in women [4, 5].

Patellar fractures are rare in children because the patella is largely cartilaginous and has greater mobility compared to adults [6]. Of all patellar fractures, less than 2 % occur in the skeletally immature patients.

Only a third of the patellar fractures encountered in the emergency department require a surgical intervention [7].

1.2 Traumatic Mechanism

Patellar fractures can result from direct and indirect forces or a combined mechanism.

The majority of patella fractures occur from a direct trauma to the front of the knee [8], for example, a fall from a height, a blow to the patella from a direct fall, or a motor vehicle crash. Usually the trauma occurs onto the flexed knee. A direct trauma may produce an incomplete, simple, or comminuted fracture. Displacement is typically minimal owing to preservation of the medial and lateral retinaculum expansion. Abrasions over the area or open injuries are common. Active knee extension may be preserved.

S. Zaffagnini (✉) • F. Raggi • A. Grassi
T. Roberti di Sarsina • C. Signorelli • M. Marcacci
Laboratorio di Biomeccanica e Innovazione
Tecnologica, Istituto Ortopedico Rizzoli,
Via Di Barbiano 1/10, 40136, Bologna (BO), Italy
e-mail: stefano.zaffagnini@unibo.it

© Springer International Publishing Switzerland 2016
F. Castoldi, D.E. Bonasia (eds.), *Fractures Around the Knee*, Fracture Management Joint by Joint,
DOI 10.1007/978-3-319-28806-2_1

Indirect mechanism is secondary to forcible eccentric quadriceps contraction while the knee is in a semiflexed position. The intrinsic strength of the patella is exceeded by the pull of the musculotendinous and ligamentous structures. Indirect injuries occur from a near fall or a stumble. The injury usually results in a transverse fracture with some inferior pole comminution and the fragment displacement is dependent on the amount of damage to the quadriceps retinaculum. Active knee extension is lost in the majority of cases.

Combined mechanism may be caused by a direct and indirect injury to the knee, such as in a fall from a height. Combined injury can present with soft tissue trauma and large fragment displacement.

1.3   Clinical Examination

The diagnosis of a patella fracture is made by collecting a complete history of the injury, performing a physical examination, and obtaining appropriate radiographic studies [9].

Patients typically present with limited or no ambulatory capacity, decreased strength, pain, swelling, and tenderness of the involved knee. A large hemarthrosis can develop from a patella fracture, especially when a large retinaculum tear is associated.

Palpation of the subcutaneous patella can demonstrate the point of maximal tenderness, and, if the displacement is significant, the physician can palpate a defect between the fragments. In nondisplaced fractures clinical examination can only demonstrate tenderness with little or no swelling.

Any major contusion, abrasion, or blister should be carefully examined to rule out an open fracture, because these constitute a surgical urgency and require surgical debridement within 6–8 h. Delays in treatment can lead to infection of the fracture site and knee joint. A simple test by the injection of more than 100 ml of saline into the knee is useful to determine if there is communication between the joint and the soft tissue injury [10].

In closed fractures, removal of the hemarthrosis decreases the intra-articular pressure, and an intra-articular injection of local anesthetic can be performed to decrease the pain and facilitate the evaluation of the extensor mechanism.

The damage to the extensor mechanism is tested by asking the patient to fully extend the leg with a pillow placed under the affected knee. Full active extension against gravity only indicates an intact extension mechanism but does not rule out the presence of a fracture. The inability to extend the knee in the presence of a patella fracture indicates a tear of both medial and lateral retinacula [1]. Testing the efficiency of the extensor mechanism is critical to determine whether a fracture will require closed or operative treatment.

Full active or passive range of motion of the knee should not be performed until a radiographic study is taken, because this can potentially further damage the retinaculum or displace the fracture.

Associated lower extremity injuries may be present in the setting of high-energy trauma. The physician must carefully evaluate the ipsilateral hip, femur, tibia, and ankle.

After completion of the clinical examination, the lower extremity is splinted in extension or slight flexion.

1.4   Imaging and Preoperative Work-Up

Radiographic studies of the patella fractures include standard x-rays of the knee in anteroposterior (AP) and lateral views and patellar views, computed tomography, and bone scanning.

Comparison views of the contralateral knee may help define the bony anatomy and soft tissue alignment, for the preoperative planning.

In the AP view, the patella normally projects onto the midline of the femoral sulcus. Its apex is located just above a line drawn across the distal profile of the femoral condyles. In the AP view, the patella is difficult to evaluate, because of the superimposition of the distal femoral condyles.

The lateral view provides a profile of the patella, fracture fragment displacement, and congruity of the articular surface. This view must be examined for fracture lines, fracture displacement, and patella height abnormalities. The proximal tibia must be visible to exclude bony avulsions of the patellar tendon from the tibial tuberosity. A "patella baja" may be indicative of a quadriceps tendon rupture, while a "patella alta" may be the sign of a patellar tendon rupture. The best way to recognize an abnormal position of the patella is the Insall-Salvati method [11]. This technique uses the ratio between the greatest diagonal patella length and the patellar tendon length. This ratio is normally around 1. A ratio < 1 suggests a high-riding patella ("patella alta") or patellar tendon rupture.

The 30° Merchant view is obtained with 45° of knee flexion and the central beam directed caudally at a 30° angle from horizontal. If a longitudinal or an osteochondral fracture is suspected, the Merchant view can be helpful.

Tendon rupture, patellar dislocation, and growth abnormality (bipartite patella) must be ruled out by imaging.

Isolated rupture of the quadriceps or patellar tendon must be excluded by clinical evaluation and by the lateral x-ray view that may indicate an abnormal position of the patella.

Dislocation, most common on the lateral side, may result in an osteochondral shear fracture with lesion of the medial margin of the patella.

The AP radiograph may demonstrate bipartite or tripartite patella, resulting from failure of fusion of two or more ossification centers. This abnormality has usually one or two fragments in the superior lateral patellar pole, with irregular, rounded, and sclerotic margins. Bipartite patella is bilateral in 50 % of cases.

Computed tomography scan may be used to better delineate fracture patterns and free osteochondral fragments or evaluate articular incongruity in case of nonunion, malunion, and patellofemoral malalignment.

Bone scintigraphy with Tc-99m can be helpful in the diagnosis of stress fractures, while indium-111 leukocyte scintigraphy can reveal infection.

1.5   Classification

The majority of patella fracture classifications use descriptive terms of the fracture pattern or location.

The Orthopaedic Trauma Association (OTA) classification system is widely accepted for the classification of patellar fractures [12]. In the OTA classification each fracture type has a code, consisting of three elements (Fig. 1.1). The first number identifies the bone (34 for the patella), and the first letter (A, B, C) describes three different fracture types:

A. Extra-articular, extensor mechanism disrupted
B. Partial articular, extensor mechanism intact, often vertical fractures
C. Complete articular, extensor mechanism disrupted

The two following numbers describe the location of the fracture and the number of fragments.

Patella fractures can be classified also in geometric terms (Fig. 1.2) such as transverse, stellate or comminute, longitudinal or marginal, proximal, or distal pole [13].

1.6   Indications

The choice of the treatment depends on the type of fracture and clinical presentation. Fractures of the patella can be treated conservatively or surgically [14].

Surgery should be avoided in patients with high preoperative risk or joint ankylosis and prior failed extensor mechanism or in nonambulatory patients [15].

Nonoperative treatment is possible in case of closed, non-displaced fractures with an intact extensor mechanism (34-B). Conservative treatment should meet the indications of fragment separation of less than 3 mm and articular incongruity less than 2 mm [12, 15].

Conservative management involves immobilization of the knee in nearly full extension for 5–6 weeks through the use of a long-leg plaster cast or a brace. The patient is allowed to partially weight-bear using crutches, advancing to full weight bearing with crutches as tolerated. Quadriceps exercise with straight-leg raising and isometric strengthening exercises should be started within a few days from the injury.

After radiographic evidence of healing, progressive active flexion and extension strengthening exercises are begun with a hinged knee brace initially locked in extension for ambulation.

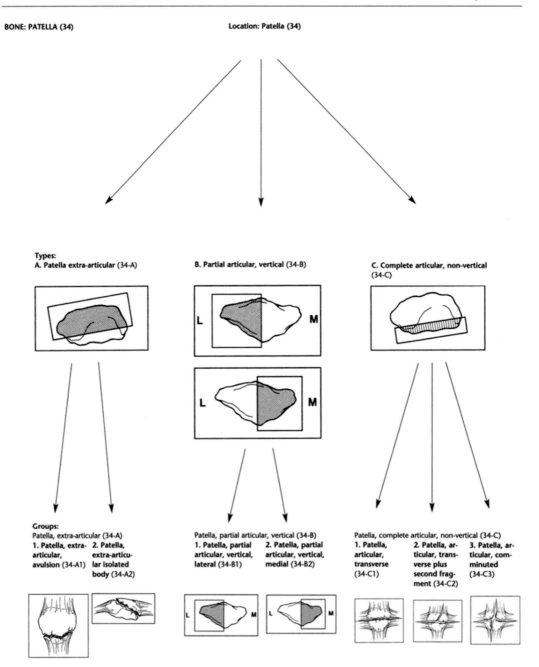

BONE: PATELLA (34)   Location: Patella (34)

Types:
A. Patella extra-articular (34-A)   **B. Partial articular, vertical (34-B)**   **C. Complete articular, non-vertical (34-C)**

Groups:
Patella, extra-articular (34-A)
1. Patella, extra-   2. Patella,
articular,   extra-articu-
avulsion (34-A1)   lar isolated
                        body (34-A2)

Patella, partial articular, vertical (34-B)
1. Patella, partial   2. Patella, partial
articular, vertical,   articular, vertical,
lateral (34-B1)   medial (34-B2)

Patella, complete articular, non-vertical (34-C)
1. Patella,   2. Patella, ar-   3. Patella, ar-
articular,   ticular, trans-   ticular, com-
transverse   verse plus   minuted
(34-C1)   second frag-   (34-C3)
                 ment (34-C2)

Note for patella:
• There are no subgroups of A.

Fig. 1.1 The OTA classification of patella fractures

Operative treatment is recommended in patella fractures with more than 2 mm of articular displacement or 3 mm of fragment separation. Indications for operative treatment also include fractures with disruption of the extensor mechanism (34-A), comminuted fractures with

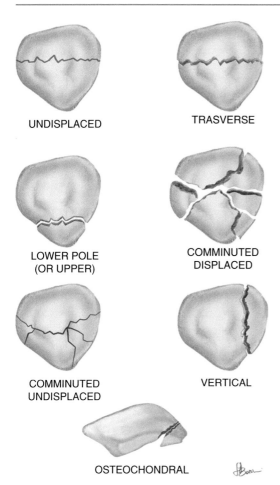

UNDISPLACED

TRASVERSE

LOWER POLE
(OR UPPER)

COMMINUTED
DISPLACED

COMMINUTED
UNDISPLACED

VERTICAL

OSTEOCHONDRAL

Fig. 1.2 Rockwood's patella fracture classification

restoring the articular surface or achieving a stable fixation is impossible.

Total patellectomy is reserved for extensive and severely comminuted fractures or as a salvage procedure for failed surgical repairs and chronic infections [14].

1.7 Surgical Technique

The goals of surgery are to preserve patella function, restore the extensor mechanism, and reduce the complications related to articular fractures.

1.7.1 Patient Position

The patient is placed supine on a radiolucent table. A cushion under the patient's ipsilateral hip is helpful to rotate the leg internally. A tourniquet around the thigh, inflated to about 200 mmHg, is used. The surgeon has to take into account that the inflated tourniquet can complicate the reduction of the fracture by retracting the quadriceps. To avoid this, the knee should be carefully flexed beyond 90° and the patella manually pushed distally to gain as much length as necessary before the tourniquet is inflated. In some cases, deflating the tourniquet while reducing the fracture can be helpful.

disruption of the articular surface (34-C), osteochondral fractures with loose bodies, and marginal or longitudinal fractures with comminution or displacement (34-B1.2/34-B2.2) [8, 12, 15].

Surgical treatment generally entails reducing the displaced fragments and fixing these together with a combination of screws, pins, and wires. Multiple methods of surgical management have been described, including tension band wire fixation, cannulated screws combined with a figure-of-eight wire, plate and screw fixation, and cerclage wiring/suturing.

Two alternative options are partial and complete patellectomy. Indications for partial patellectomy are limited but include the presence of a large, salvageable fragment in the presence of a smaller, comminuted polar fragment, where

1.7.2 Surgical Approach

Several surgical approaches have been described for the operative treatment of patella fractures.

The most common approach is a midline longitudinal incision over the patella that can be extended proximally or distally (Fig. 1.3).

Parapatellar incisions are also possible; these are indicated in case of open fractures where the skin lesion is incorporated into the approach.

The transverse approach should be avoided in order not to damage the infrapatellar branch of the saphenous nerve.

After incision of the superficial fascia, the extensor apparatus is exposed and tears in the auxiliary extensors can be identified. If a knee

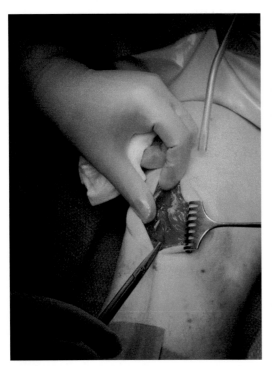

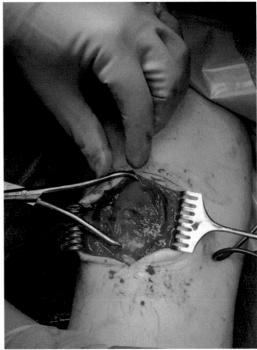

Fig. 1.3 Surgical approach and exposure of the patella

Fig. 1.4 Reduction technique using pointed bone reduction forceps

joint inspection is necessary, a medial parapatellar arthrotomy is made. Intra-articular procedures can be performed as needed. In case of open fractures or a preexisting chronic bursitis, the prepatellar bursa may be excised; this is normally not required in closed fractures.

1.7.3 Reduction and Fixation Techniques

As in all articular fractures, surgical treatment begins with achieving an accurate reduction of the articular surface. The larger fragments are reduced using a large pointed bone reduction forceps (Fig. 1.4). In type A or C fractures, reduction is easier in a full or hyperextended position of the knee. Longitudinal type B fractures are sometimes better reduced with the knee flexed. A temporary Kirschner wire fixation is often used in comminuted fractures. The wires can also be used as joysticks to help in reducing the fragments. Anatomical reduction of the articular surface is monitored by palpating the joint from inside with the knee fully extended or slightly hyperextended. This digital palpation of the articular surface is normally possible through tears or incisions in the medial or lateral retinaculum.

1.7.3.1 Tension Band Wiring

The principle of this technique is to convert the tension force into compression force as the knee is flexed. The patella is loaded in tension by the extension mechanism. In fractured patellae this causes displacement of the fragments. Proper application of a tension band wire construct to a patella fracture converts this tension force into compression at the level of the articular surface.

The tension band wire construct alone is generally reserved for the displaced transverse patella fracture.

Two parallel Kirschner wires (1.6–2 mm) are placed longitudinally, through the reduced fragments. The ideal level for the pins lies in the center of the patella, approximately 5 mm below its anterior surface.

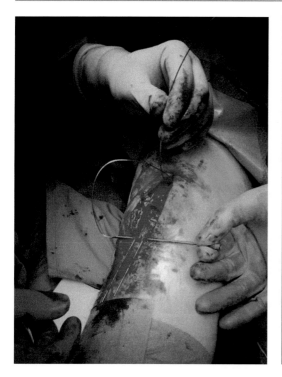

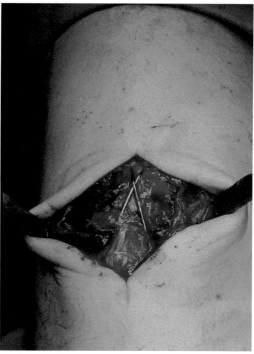

Fig. 1.5 Passage of the cerclage at the inferior pole using a cannula

Fig. 1.6 The figure-of-eight wire correctly positioned

A sufficiently long (about 30 cm), 1.0- or 1.25-mm-thick cerclage wire is then passed in a figure-of-eight way, adjacent to the inferior and superior poles and posterior to the parallel K-wires. The wire should be as close as possible to the bone throughout its whole course. A curved large bore needle or cannula can be helpful to pass the cerclage wires through the ligamentous structures (patellar and quadriceps tendons) and around the K-wires close to the bone (Fig. 1.5). The figure-of-eight wire must not lie on top of the quadriceps or patellar tendons, because the tightening of the wire can result in necrosis of the underlying tendon (Fig. 1.6) [16].

While tightening the cerclage with the knee in extension, the reduction is checked by palpating the retropatellar surface. After tightening the cerclage, the proximal pin ends will be bent, shortened, and turned toward the quadriceps tendon and driven into the patella to prevent soft tissue irritation and loosening. The distal pin ends are only trimmed, not bent, for easier removal.

In comminuted fractures, with many small fragments, the tension band technique must be combined with an additional circumferential cerclage around the fractured patella (Fig. 1.7). The placement of this cerclage should be the initial step of stabilization to avoid further displacement as tension band wiring is performed.

1.7.3.2 Tension Banding plus Lag Screws

In transverse fractures, the two main fragments are often further fragmented in halves or thirds. The minor fragments are generally reduced and fixed in order to end up with two main fragments that can be fixed with the tension band technique. Tension band wiring is possible only if the two main fragments have been reconstructed by lag screws. After reduction of fragments and temporary fixation by a pointed reduction forceps, 3.5 mm cortex screws are implanted. After fixation of the fragments, a tension band wire construct can be performed. This type of construct can be challenging, as the interfragmentary screws may interfere with the Kirschner wire of the

Fig. 1.7 (**a**) A comminuted displaced patella fracture. (**b**) Stabilization with a tension band wire combined with an additional circumferential cerclage

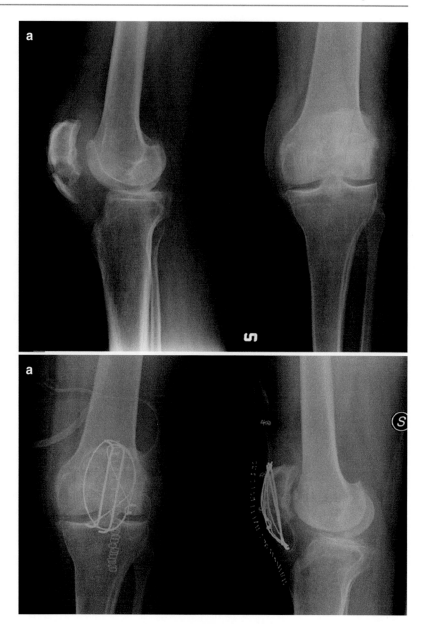

tension band. To avoid this problem, the screws are placed close to the retropatellar surface, leaving enough space for the K-wires. When the fragments are too small to be fixed with a screw, 1.6 mm K-wires can be used.

Patellar pole fractures are best stabilized by lag screws and an additional tension band wiring to neutralize bending forces.

Osteochondral fractures can be treated with a screw, a K-wire, or both (Fig. 1.8).

1.7.3.3 Partial and Total Patellectomy

With highly comminuted fractures involving a substantial amount of the patella, partial patellectomy may be considered. Partial patellectomy is preferred to total patellectomy, whenever possible, as it keeps the lever arm intact. Partial patellectomy is a technique primarily reserved for fractures of the extreme inferior and superior poles of the patella. Essentially, the bony fragments are excised, and the quadriceps tendon or

Fig. 1.8 (**a**) An osteochondral fracture of the superomedial corner of the patella. (**b**) Stabilization of the fragment with a screw and a K-wire

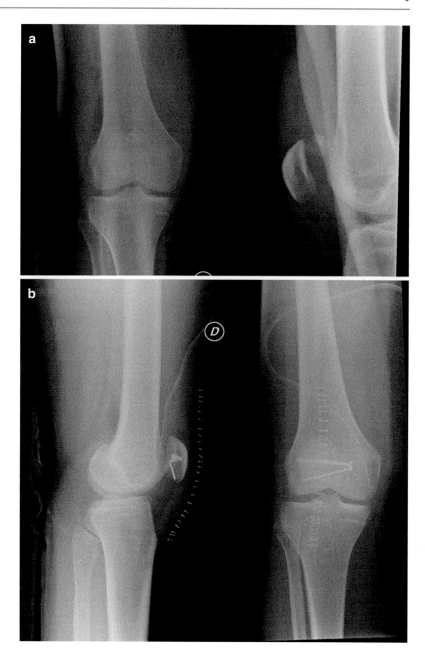

the patella ligament is advanced to the fracture bed. Repair can be performed with heavy braided suture passed through transosseous tunnels.

If the comminuted area is in the middle of the patella, an osteotomy can be done proximally and distally in order to remove the comminuted part. Reduction and fixation are then performed, as in a transverse fracture can be done.

Currently, total patellectomy for the treatment of acute patellar fracture is generally not recommended. Substantial weakness of the extensor mechanism has been demonstrated in total patellectomy patients [17].

In case of severe comminution or failed surgical repair, patellectomy may be the only way to manage the injury. All bony fragments and damaged tissue are removed by sharp dissection leaving as much extensor apparatus as possible. Tendinous reconstruction then follows. A gap of 3–4 cm can be treated by direct suture. Shortening of the extensor apparatus is beneficial as it increases the muscle preload. If a direct suture is impossible, an advancement of the vastus medialis obliquus to cover the longitudinal defect left after patellectomy has been advocated to promote healing and to preserve strength of the extensor mechanism [18].

1.8   Postoperative Regimen

The stability of the fracture repair dictates the course of postoperative regimen and rehabilitation. With a stable fixation early active range-of-motion exercises and partial to full weight bearing in hinged knee brace can be allowed. When the patient is walking, a knee brace locked in extension is recommended. This may reduce the force of the extensor mechanism across the repair.

Drains are removed on the first or second postoperative day, depending on the amount of wound drainage. Then the patient begins with isometric exercises and mobilization. Partial weight bearing from 15 kg to half of the body weight for 6 weeks and active assisted motion from full extension to 90° of flexion are allowed, after wound healing. With radiographic evidence of fracture healing at 4–6 weeks, resistive exercises may be started. Gradual weaning off the brace should occur over the next 3–6 months, and return to sport or vigorous activities should not occur until rehabilitation is complete at 4–6 months.

In case of comminuted fractures with unstable fixation, an immobilization using a long-leg cast or knee brace locked in extension is required. Active and passive flexion exercises should be delayed until radiographic evidence of healing.

1.9   Complications

1.9.1   Disturbed Wound Healing

The optimal plane of tissue dissection lies between the subcutaneous fascia and the extensor apparatus. In order to preserve the blood supply to the skin and avoid necrosis of the wound margins, the subcutaneous tissue must not be separated from the skin. Improper use of skin retractors can also result in such problems.

1.9.2   Deep Infection

The rate of infection for patella fractures is low in most case series. The rate of infection of open patella fractures is 10.7 % [19].

Postoperative wound infection should be recognized and treated according to standard protocols.

Revision with debridement and irrigation is indicated every other day until wound healing is secured. Stable fixation may be retained with an aggressive surgical debridement and the use of intravenous antibiotics. Areas of infected bone should undergo aggressive removal of all nonviable tissue. With deep infection, long-term culture-specific antibiotic application (6 weeks) is recommended.

1.9.3   Implant-Related Irritation

One major disadvantage of the tension wire technique is painful hardware. This problem is very common and is related to irritation of the capsule and tendons. Intraoperatively the surgeon should pay special attention to place prominent hardware into the bone and surrounding soft tissues to prevent painful implants.

1.9.4   Implant Failure

With the use of early aggressive range-of-motion exercises, re-displacement of the fracture fragments can occur due to inadequate fixation or postoperative immobilization.

Implant failure requires a revision only if the main fragments are displaced or the articular surface is showing incongruity. A common complication is proximal K-wire migration. To prevent this, the wire ends should be bent to a loop and the tension band wire is then pulled through the two proximal loops holding the K-wires in stable position [20].

1.9.5 Loss of Motion

Functional range of motion can usually be achieved with stable internal fixation and early aggressive physical therapy.

In case of limited flexion, intensive physiotherapy is indicated. Failure of conservative treatment is an indication for a controlled manipulation under anesthesia. If the range of motion does not improve with closed arthrolysis, an arthroscopic arthrolysis will be the next step, removing scar contractions from the upper recess. After the arthroscopic treatment aggressive physical therapy should be started.

1.9.6 Posttraumatic Arthritis

Osteoarthritis with patellofemoral pain may be the late complication of a patella fracture. There are few reports regarding knee arthrosis after patella fracture [4, 21]. Radiographic signs of knee arthritis after patella fracture are evident in approximately 50 % of patients in a long-term follow-up.

1.10 Results

Comparing the various outcome-based studies after a patellar fracture is difficult. Most studies demonstrated reliable healing after patella fracture fixation or reported subjective outcomes.

Two recent case series have been published. Le Brun et al. prospectively examined a series of 40 patella fractures at 1 year of follow-up, showing poor outcomes [22]. It has been shown that one-third of the patients with retained implants reported periodic implant irritation and more than 50 % of the patients required implant removal. Approximately 20 % of the patients had an extensor lag of at least 5°. A decreased extension strength was also noted.

In the second study, a clinical series of 50 patella fractures were evaluated at 6 and 12 months of follow-up and compared with 50 quadriceps or patellar tendon ruptures. At 12-month follow-up, there were no significant differences between the two study groups with respect to knee range of motion, Tegner, radiographic arthritis, Lysholm, and SF-36 scores. In the patella fracture group, the thigh circumference was significantly smaller [23].

There are few reports regarding knee arthritis after patella fracture. Sorensen reported 10–30-year outcomes of 64 patients with patella fracture (22 patients treated operatively); approximately 55 % of surgically treated and 69 % of nonoperatively treated patients were symptom free (no significant difference) [21]. Radiographic changes consistent with patellofemoral arthrosis were noted in 45 of the 64 patients, and 21 patients were symptomatic. In another report of 40 patella fractures at 30-year follow-up, all patients showed reduction of the lateral patellofemoral joint space (more severe in the case of fracture gap or incongruity), consistent with arthrosis, but only 14 patients (35 %) had subjective complaints [24]. In a series of 40 patients treated with partial patellectomy for patella fracture, good-to-excellent results were noted in 77.5 % of the patients (31 patients), and 52.5 % (21 patients) were noted to have patellofemoral arthrosis on plain radiographs [25].

References

1. Bostrom A (1972) Fracture of the patella: a study of 422 patellar fractures. Acta Orthop Scand 143:1–80
2. Springorum HP, Siewe J, Dargel J, Schiffer G, Michael JW, Eysel P (2011) Classification and treatment of patella fractures. Orthopade 40(10):877–880
3. Court-Brown CM, Caesar B (2006) Epidemiology of adult fractures: a review. Injury 37(8):691–697
4. Nummi J (1971) Fracture of the patella: a clinical study of 707 patellar fractures. Ann Chir Gynaecol Fenn 179:1–85
5. Nummi J (1971) Operative treatment of patellar fractures. Acta Orthop Scand 42:437–438
6. Zionts LE (2002) Fractures around the knee in children. J Am Acad Orthop Surg 10(5):345–355, Review
7. Scilaris TA, Grantham JL, Prayson MJ, Marshall MP, Hamilton JJ, Williams JL (1998) Biomechanical

comparison of fixation methods in transverse patella fractures. J Orthop Trauma 12:356–359

8. Muller M, Allgower M, Schneider R, Willenegger H (1991) Manual of internal fixation: techniques recommended by the AO-ASIF group, 3rd edn. Springer, Berlin

9. Helfet DL, Haas NP, Schatzker J, Matter P, Moser R, Hanson B (2003) AO philosophy and principles of fracture management-its evolution and evaluation. J Bone Joint Surg Am Vol 85(6):1156–1160

10. Nord RM, Quach T, Walsh M, Pereira D, Tejwani NC (2009) Detection of traumatic arthrotomy of the knee using the saline solution load test. J Bone Joint Surg Am 91(1):66–70

11. Insall J, Salvati E (1971) Patella position in the normal knee joint. Radiology 101(1):101–104

12. Fracture and Dislocation Classification Compendium at http://www.ota.org/compendium/compendium.html

13. Bucholz RW, Heckman JD, Court-Brown C et al (eds) (2006) Rockwood and Green's fractures in adults, 6th edn. Lippincott Williams & Wilkins, Philadelphia

14. Insall JN, Scott WN (2006) Surgery of the knee, vol 2, 4th edn. Churchill Livingstone, New York

15. Melvin JS, Mehta S (2011) Patella fractures in adults. J Am Acad Orthop Surg 19(4):198–207

16. Della Rocca GJ (2013) Displaced patella fractures. J Knee Surg 26(5):293–299.doi:10.1055/s-0033-1353988, Epub 2013 Aug 21

17. Lennox IA, Cobb AG, Knowles J, Bentley G (1994) Knee function after patellectomy. A 12- to 48- year follow up. J Bone Joint Surg Br 76(3):485–487

18. Günal I, Taymaz A, Köse N, Göktürk E, Seber S (1997) Patellectomy with vastus medialis obliquus advancement for comminuted patellar fractures: a prospective randomised trial. J Bone Joint Surg Br 79(1):13–16

19. Torchia ME, Lewallen DG (1996) Open fractures of the patella. J Orthop Trauma 10:403–409

20. Us AK, Kinik H (1966) Self locking tension band technique in transverse patellar fractures. Int Orthop 20:357–358

21. Sorensen KH (1964) The late prognosis after fracture of the patella. Acta Orthop Scand 34:198–212

22. LeBrun CT, Langford JR, Sagi HC (2012) Functional outcomes after operatively treated patella fractures. J Orthop Trauma 26(7):422–426

23. Tejwani NC, Lekic N, Bechtel C, Montero N, Egol KA (2012) Outcomes after knee joint extensor mechanism disruptions: is better to fracture the patella or rupture the tendon? J Orthop Trauma 26(11):648–651

24. Edwards B, Johnell O, Redlund-Johnell I (1989) Patellar fractures. A 30-year follow-up. Acta Orthop Scand 60(6):712–714

25. Saltzman CL, Goulet JA, McClellan RT, Schneider LA, Matthews LS (1990) Results of treatment of displaced patellar fractures by partial patellectomy. J Bone Joint Surg Am 72(9):1279–1285

Tibial Eminence Fractures

Jessica Hanley and Annunziato Amendola

Abstract

Tibial intercondylar eminence fractures are relatively rare and occur with an estimated incidence of 3 in 100,000 people every year. These injuries are much less common than intrasubstance tears of the anterior cruciate ligament (ACL), especially in adults. Tibial spine fractures represent a difficult problem but are important to recognize and manage appropriately. This chapter discusses non-operative and operative management of these injuries, as well as patient outcomes and potential complications of treatment. Surgical technique, using open and arthroscopic methods with both screw and suture fixation, is also described.

2.1 Epidemiology

Tibial intercondylar eminence fractures were first described by A. Poncet in 1875. He described them quite accurately as "a tearing off of the spine of the tibia by the anterior cruciate ligament" [1]. Also referred to as tibial spine fractures, these are relatively rare injuries and occur with an estimated incidence of 3 in 100,000 people every year [2, 3]. Most commonly, these fractures happen in skeletally immature individuals between the ages of 8 and 14 years, but can occur at any age [4–7]. These injuries are much less common than intrasubstance tears of the anterior cruciate ligament (ACL), especially in adults. Furthermore, studies have shown that up to 40 % are associated with concomitant injuries to the meniscus, collaterals, and retinacular or articular cartilage [8–10]. Tibial spine fractures represent a difficult problem, as most orthopedic surgeons and sports medicine physician specialists have infrequent experience with these injuries. They are important to recognize and manage appropriately due to the possible detrimental functional outcomes if left untreated in a displaced position.

2.2 Traumatic Mechanism

Tibial eminence fractures traditionally occur with higher-energy mechanisms such as cycling or skiing accidents, motor vehicle collisions, or contact sports including football, soccer, or rugby [11–14]. Most patients describe falling on a bent knee causing an internal twisting moment of the tibia on the femur, similar to the moment force required to cause an ACL tear [5, 15]. This condition is most common in the skeletally immature population because the tibial eminence is not completely ossified. Energy is transferred through the knee, and failure occurs

J. Hanley, MD (✉) • A. Amendola, MD
Department of Orthopaedic Surgery, University of Iowa, Iowa City, IA, USA

© Springer International Publishing Switzerland 2016
F. Castoldi, D.E. Bonasia (eds.), *Fractures Around the Knee*, Fracture Management Joint by Joint,
DOI 10.1007/978-3-319-28806-2_2

through the cartilage rather than rupturing the tough ligamentous structures [10]. Although many of these fractures occur without concomitant ACL rupture, the amount of force transferred through the ACL can cause attenuation of the ligament and ultimately lead to clinical instability [16, 17].

It is important to understand the anatomy and biomechanics of the knee when managing eminence fractures. The tibial spine is critical in the biomechanical functioning of the ACL. The ACL begins 10–14 mm behind the anterior border of the tibia and extends to the medial and lateral tibial eminence [10]. The ACL, as well as the ligamentous attachments of the medial and lateral menisci, inserts separately on the tibial eminence. Thus, a fracture through the tibial spine can effectively act like an ACL rupture. The blood supply travels through the ACL from the middle geniculate artery and is not normally disrupted. Accordingly, osteonecrosis of the fracture fragment is not typically seen with these injuries [10].

2.3   Clinical Examination

The classic patient with a tibial eminence fracture presents with a high-energy mechanism, significant pain, clinical signs of instability, and an acute hemarthrosis. They are unable to bear weight and tend to hold their knee in flexion. Pain and joint swelling, rather than impingement of the avulsed piece, typically impede extension of the knee. The fracture fragment generally lies below the hollow of the intercondylar notch and does not interfere with motion; however, if it is significantly displaced, it can cause impingement.

It is important to obtain a detailed and complete history and physical exam upon presentation. Evaluation of the patient's neurovascular status and a thorough musculoskeletal examination of the knee are essential to assess the extent of injury. Importantly, associated ligamentous laxity, i.e., ACL, MCL, and PLC injuries, and possible bony or meniscal injuries about the knee must be specifically considered. The Lachman test, the anterior drawer, and the pivot shift examination are helpful in the assessment of the integrity of the ACL. However, in the acute swollen knee, pivot shift and anterior drawer testing are painful, and

therefore the Lachman test is preferred. The posterior drawer and sag sign can be useful in identifying PCL injuries. Palpation of the joint lines and varus/valgus stressing are important to rule out any other associated injuries to the knee. These tests are often difficult to perform in the acutely injured knee, but can be gently achieved for a complete exam.

2.4   Imaging and Preoperative Workup

For any patient with a suspected knee injury, AP and lateral plain films of the knee must first be obtained. These will be helpful in most cases to identify a fracture of the tibial eminence as well as rule out other bony abnormalities. It is important not to confuse fractures of the spine with fractures of the femoral condyles or inferior pole of the patella. If there is any uncertainty, especially with the skeletally immature patient, it is prudent to obtain contralateral knee films. Griffith et al. demonstrated that all tibial avulsion fractures are visible on X-ray, but advanced imaging is warranted at times to better characterize the fracture and provide useful information for preoperative planning [18]. A CT scan or MRI is not absolutely necessary but can sometimes provide details to improve decision-making and treatment plans (Fig. 2.1).

CT scan better clarifies the bony details including the amount of comminution, displacement, orientation, size, and shape as well as the extent of involvement of the tibial spine. This information can be helpful in deciding which treatment options to pursue. For example, a CT may provide the surgeon with details about whether or not the fracture fragment is large enough to be amenable to screw versus suture fixation. MRI imaging can improve the preoperative assessment of concomitant injuries in the knee, including meniscal, cartilage, and ligamentous damage, including intrasubstance ACL injury. This advanced information can dictate surgical plans, including the decision to perform ACL reconstruction versus fracture fixation. Additionally, it can detect physeal injuries in children that may otherwise be missed. Rehabilitation and ACL graft choices may also be affected by appreciating the complete injury on the MRI (Fig. 2.2).

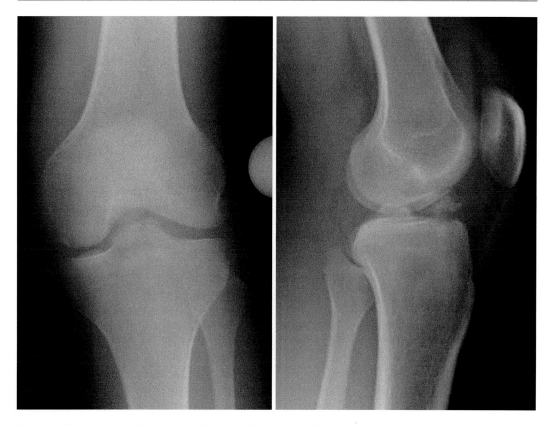

Fig. 2.1 AP and lateral radiographs of a displaced tibial eminence fracture

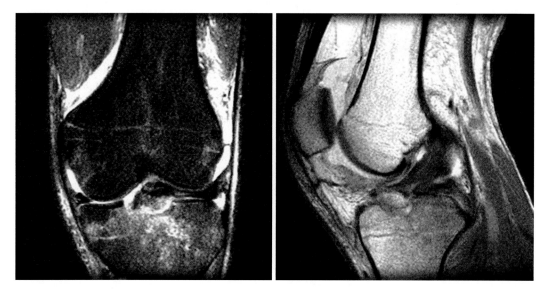

Fig. 2.2 Select MRI images of a tibial eminence fracture

2.5   Classification

The classification of tibial eminence fractures is attributed to Dr. Marvin Meyers and Dr. Francis McKeever in 1959. The Meyers and McKeever classification system was relatively simple and based on the amount of bony displacement from the tibia seen on a lateral X-ray of the knee [11]. Initially, three types of tibial spine fractures were described: Type I is defined as a nondisplaced or minimally displaced fracture with excellent bony apposition. Type II has greater displacement than type I, with the anterior half of the fragment avulsed from the bone. Type III has no bony attachment to the tibia and is essentially a complete avulsion of the tibial eminence. Zaricznyj added a fourth type of fracture to the classification system in 1977. Type IV describes a comminuted tibial spine fragment [19]. Since the original description by Meyers and McKeever, type III fractures have also been subcategorized based on the extent of the ACL footprint involvement. Lubowitz et al. described type IIIA tibial spine fracture as involving the ACL insertion only. Type IIIB includes the entire intercondylar eminence rather than just the ACL insertion [5] (Fig. 2.3; Table 2.1).

2.6   Indications

The characteristics and classification of tibial eminence fractures are important in choosing an appropriate treatment. The goals of treatment are to restore the integrity of the tibial plateau, increase stability and ACL function, eliminate any mechanical blocks caused by the injury, and ultimately improve functional capacity for the patient to pre-injury levels.

2.6.1   Nondisplaced Fractures

Nonoperative management can usually only be reserved for type I or II fractures. If tibial spine fragments are minimally displaced or nondisplaced, the associated hemarthrosis should be aspirated in the acute setting and the knee should be immobilized for a period of time, usually 4–8 weeks. The patient is traditionally placed into a long leg cast or knee immobilizer in full extension.

However, there is some controversy around the optimal degree of flexion for immobilization. Beaty and Kumar have endorsed 10–15° as an ideal position of immobilization [20]. Meyers and McKeever as well as Willis et al. have recommended 20° [11, 21]. Fyfe and Jackson proposed that since the ACL is tight in extension, 30–50° of flexion is optimal to reduce tension on the avulsed fragment [22]. Immobilization in hyperextension should be avoided as it can place unnecessary tension on the popliteal vessels putting the patient at risk of vascular disruption and/or compartment syndrome. Furthermore, subjective discomfort is intensified when a patient is casted in hyperextension.

Overall, the most important element of conservative management is anatomic or near anatomic reduction of the tibial eminence. Even though the ACL is tight in extension, the fragment best reduces in extension, not in flexion. Radiographs should be taken or fluoroscopy used to ensure acceptable alignment, which is generally defined as <3 mm of superior displacement on the lateral X-ray. Anatomic reduction of the tibial spine generally occurs in full extension; thus, the preferred method of the author is to immobilize patients in full extension.

Patients being treated with cast immobilization should be closely monitored with radiographs and clinical examination weekly or biweekly. Duration of immobilization should be governed by the evidence of radiographic union as well as patient's age and compliance with treatment. Children usually require 4–6 weeks of immobilization, while skeletally mature individuals require slightly longer, usually 6–8 weeks.

Patients should remain nonweightbearing on the affected extremity throughout the course of immobilization. Our recommendation is to begin weightbearing with active and passive knee range of motion after radiographic signs of bone healing are seen. Generally, patients will achieve pre-injury range of motion and activity levels approximately 3–4 months after the injury.

Nonoperative treatment of type II tibial eminence fractures is another point of controversy in the literature. There is debate surrounding whether or not attempt at closed reduction is useful in this

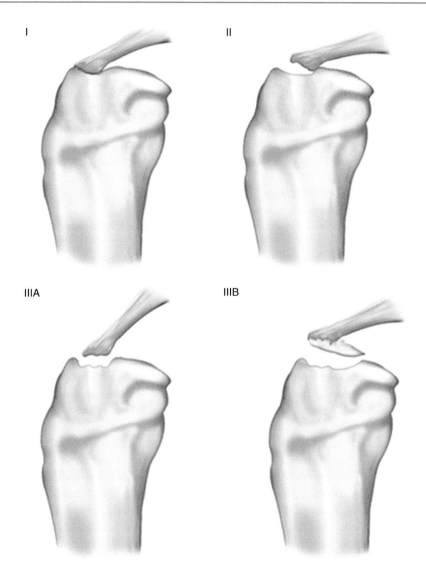

Fig. 2.3 The modified Meyers and McKeever classification system (Adapted from Lubowitz et al. [5])

Table 2.1 The modified Meyers and McKeever classification system

Type I	Type II	Type III	Type IV
◆ Good bone apposition ◆ Slight elevation of the anterior margin of the tibia	◆ Greater displacement of fragment than type I ◆ Anterior 1/3 to 1/2 of fragment is elevated from the bone ◆ Beaklike appearance on the lateral X-ray	◆ Complete avulsion of the fracture fragment ◆ No bony apposition between the tibia and fragment ◆ Fragment may be rotated ▶ *IIIA*: avulsion of ACL insertion only ▶ *IIIB*: avulsion of the entire tibial spine	◆ Significant comminution of the fracture fragment ◆ Complete avulsion injury ◆ No bony apposition of the fragment and tibia

population. Closed reduction is generally difficult and forced hyperextension can displace the fragment further. Often there is a physical block to reduction, making closed reduction difficult. Most commonly, the anterior horn of the medial meniscus becomes incarcerated in between the bone ends, preventing anatomic reduction. The lateral meniscus and intermeniscal ligament have also been reported to become interposed in the fracture. Kocher et al. reported that 26 out of 49 (53 %) skeletally immature patients with type II fractures have soft tissue interposition noted on arthroscopic investigation [9].

2.6.2 Displaced Fractures

Type III and IV fractures, as well as Type II fractures that fail closed reduction, are usually treated operatively unless the patient's condition precludes the possibility of operative intervention [19, 23, 24]. Historically, open arthrotomy and fixation was the treatment method of choice. Although more technically challenging, arthroscopic and minimally invasive techniques have become increasingly popular. Arthroscopic-assisted reduction of tibial eminence fractures was first described in 1982 by McLennan [25]. Although arthroscopy is generally preferred, the literature does not necessarily support the superiority of one technique over another. It is recommended that the surgeon approach the tibial eminence fracture by whichever method is more comfortable and familiar. Surgical technique will be discussed later in this chapter.

The ACL commonly remains intact with a tibial eminence fracture; however sometimes structural damage and laxity are seen. Instability is generally not a clinical concern for patients even if there is ligamentous damage or attenuation at the time of injury. 74 % of children at long-term follow-up had ligamentous laxity on KT-100 testing but no subjective complaints of instability [21]. There is debate regarding the necessity of ACL reconstruction and/or repair of other possibly damaged structures in the knee. ACL reconstruction is only recommended if symptomatic laxity and instability exists after healing of the tibial eminence [5, 10, 26, 27].

2.7 Surgical Technique

2.7.1 Anesthesia

Epidural, spinal, and general anesthesia are all acceptable methods of anesthesia during operative fixation of a tibial eminence fracture. The preferred method of the author is general anesthesia in children and a regional block combined general anesthetic in adults.

2.7.2 Patient Positioning

The patient should be positioned depending on the surgeon's preference and planned surgical approach.

Arthroscopic techniques are generally preferred and performed supine with the leg in arthroscopic leg holder with the end of the bed flexed or extended. The contralateral extremity is abducted away from the field to allow for a fluoroscopy machine to be utilized intraoperatively. A non-sterile tourniquet should be placed but not inflated unless absolutely necessary. Open approaches can be utilized and are often completed with the patient supine, allowing excellent visualization and manipulation of the leg. Open surgery for eminence fracture fixation is required in cases with open reduction of more extensive tibial plateau fractures or in open multi-ligament knee surgery where an eminence fracture is only part of the picture. These will not be discussed as part of this chapter.

2.7.3 Recommended Surgical Approach: Arthroscopic Reduction and Internal Fixation

2.7.3.1 Arthroscopic Reduction and Screw Fixation

Anteromedial and anterolateral standard portals can be made for visualization and diagnostic arthroscopy. An arthroscopic inspection of the entire knee should be performed prior to any fixation to look for other injuries to the cartilage or ligaments about the knee. The fracture should be freed from any obvious soft tissue interposition and debrided as is standard protocol in fixation of any fracture. Any

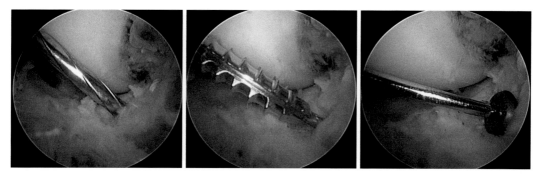

Fig. 2.4 Screw fixation of a tibial eminence fracture

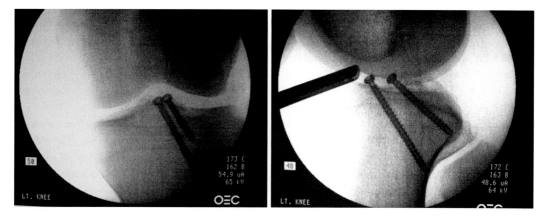

Fig. 2.5 Fluoro spots of screw fixation of a tibial eminence fracture

meniscal interposition (usually the anterior horn of the medial meniscus) can be moved out of the way with a probe to allow the anterior extent of the fracture to reduce. Adequate and anatomic reduction is imperative for an excellent outcome. Fracture reduction can and should be performed under direct visualization. The fracture, if a large single fragment, can be manipulated with a probe, grasper, or elevator into the reduced position. Once the fracture is reducible and the decision for screw fixation has been made, a third anterior mid-medial patellar portal can be made. With the scope in the lateral portal, and the fracture held reduced through the medial portal, a temporary K-wire or guide wire for a 3.5 or 4 mm screw can be inserted from the mid-medial patellar portal. Fluoroscopy can be utilized to confirm reduction and fixation.

Once the fracture has been adequately reduced, a cannulated drill and one or two screws can be inserted through the mid-medial patellar portal screw. With screw fixation, the fracture

fragment should be at least three times the size of the screw diameter to prevent disruption of the fragment [28]. Alternatively, suture fixation may be utilized depending on the fracture pattern and surgeon preference. Screw fixation has limited utility in the comminuted type IV fracture where adequate bony purchase may be challenging (Figs. 2.4 and 2.5).

2.7.3.2 Arthroscopic Reduction and Suture Fixation

If the fracture fragment is small or fragmented and the ACL is in good structural condition, repair is still indicated versus ACL reconstruction or augmentation. Suture fixation techniques can be advantageous in these situations, and the technique has been described with several variations over the years [8, 27, 29–33]. For suture repair, an ACL drill guide, 2.4 mm smooth guide wires, an arthroscopic suturing device, and a suture passing device are required.

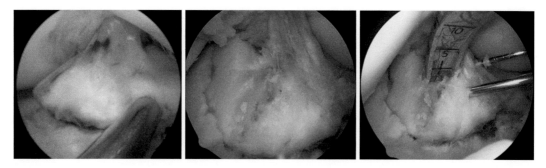

Fig. 2.6 Arthroscopic reduction of tibial eminence fracture

With the fragment reduced or reducible (a K-wire can be used to hold the fragment in place while inserting sutures as in the technique above), through the medial portal, insert the ACL guide and drill 2 x 2.4 guide wires just anterior to the fragment(s). Remove one guide wire and insert a suture passer through this 2.4 drill hole into the joint.

Through the medial portal, grasp the base of the ACL tissue with nonabsorbable suture and pull the suture through the bone tunnel with the suture passer. Repeat the same routine with the other guide wire tunnel. The second suture can be placed from the lateral portal and exchange the arthroscope into the medial portal for viewing.

These two sutures can be tied over a bone bridge anteriorly on the tibia or over a button if desired. Direct visualization of the ACL being cinched down into its base when tying the sutures confirms reduction and tensioning. Additional sutures can be placed if necessary for additional fixation.

2.7.3.3 Screw Versus Suture Fixation

Biomechanical studies have looked at the strength of fixation with sutures and screws in direct comparison. Bong et al. and Eggers et al. have suggested that suture fixation has greater fixation strength during cyclic loading when compared with screw fixation [34, 35]. Both studies suggested that fiberwire had the highest ultimate biomechanical strength and load to failure when compared to screw fixation. Eggers et al. also suggest that adding a second screw to a screw construct does not improve fixation strength [35].

Tsukada et al. suggest antegrade screw fixation is slightly superior in resisting cyclic loading forces when compared to retrograde screw or suture fixation [36]. Mahar et al. show no superiority of suture versus screw fixation and suggest that both are acceptable methods of fixation [37]. Overall, cadaveric studies seem to suggest that there is limited, if any, superiority of either method of fixation. Functional outcomes also appear to be equivalent [26]. Nevertheless, it is worth noting that screw fixation has a higher rate of reoperation for removal of prominent and irritating hardware. It is most important that the surgeon be comfortable with arthroscopic technique so that stable fixation can be achieved (Fig. 2.6).

2.7.4 Open Reduction Internal Fixation

For an open approach, an incision is made just medial to the midline from the distal pole of the patella down toward the tuberosity. An arthrotomy just medial to the patellar tendon is performed after careful soft tissue dissection. The patellar tendon and patella are retracted laterally to expose the fat pad. Portions of the fat pad may be excised to improve visibility of the tibial plateau and eminence. Care must be taken to inspect and protect the menisci and intermeniscal ligament. These may be damaged or interposed in the fracture site. Identification of injury or incarceration is imperative to allow anatomic reduction. Fixation techniques can be the same as the arthroscopic with either screw fixation or suture repair through small drill holes.

2.8 Postoperative Regimen

Regardless of the method of fixation—open or arthroscopic with suture or screw fixation—it is of utmost importance to initiate early range of motion after surgery. Patients with surgical fixation of their tibial spine are at high risk of developing limitations of knee motion. Patients are hesitant to aggressively range their knee through a complete cycle because of pain and fear of reinjury. If extensive scar forms due to inadequate rehabilitation, these patients may have permanent flexion deformities or require additional surgeries for arthrofibrosis [30, 38, 39].

Weightbearing status and immobilization are largely based on the nature of the fracture and fracture type, as well as the quality of fixation and patient compliance. These are difficult variables to control so postoperative regimen must be individualized. Type I fractures managed nonoperatively are generally treated with cast immobilization and nonweightbearing for 4 weeks in children and 6 weeks in adults. After this, gentle range of motion and protected weightbearing are begun. Patients with operatively fixed fractures are generally placed into a knee immobilizer or cast locked in extension for 2 weeks, and range of motion is initiated early to prevent stiffness in the knee. Depending on the type and stability of fixation, weightbearing status may differ. However, most patients remain nonweightbearing for the first 2 weeks after surgery and are slowly transitioned to weightbearing as tolerated.

2.9 Complications

Although rare, complications can occur after tibial spine fracture fixation and are worth discussing. Loss of fixation and hardware irritation are significant problems after operative intervention. Loss of fixation may result in malunion or nonunion. Patients with this complication experience residual pain, laxity and instability in the knee,

impaired range of motion, and impingement. Both malunion and nonunion are uncommon but can be devastating. Significant malunion can result in impingement in terminal extension leading to loss of 5–10° of extension, accompanied by anterior knee pain. Repeat surgery may have a chance of salvaging such complications. In minor cases, surgical debridement may be adequate [40–42]. In major malunions or nonunions, revision fixation and reduction with or without bone grafting may be necessary [43, 44].

Fixation failure may also lead to chondral damage from hardware irritation. These complications are avoidable if proper technique is utilized. Limiting fixation to one or two screws that are no more than 4 mm diameter can decrease hardware complications. Countersinking screws or using headless screws is also advised in order to avoid prominent hardware. For comminuted fractures, suture fixation is recommended as loss of fixation can occur without adequate bone stock and screw purchase. Notably, a higher reoperation rate has been noted with screw fixation than with suture fixation [4].

ACL laxity or knee instability is also a possible complication after repair of a tibial spine fracture. Many patients, including up to 74 % of children, have objective laxity but do not report subjective instability [16]. This laxity is generally treated nonoperatively unless it becomes symptomatic. If symptomatic, the patient may elect to undergo surgical reconstruction of the ACL [5, 10, 26, 27].

Knee stiffness is another complication of both operative and nonoperative management. Up to 60 % of patients with a tibial spine fracture may experience knee stiffness, usually resulting in a loss of approximately 5–10° of terminal extension. This can be avoided with anatomic reduction and appropriate initiation of range of motion protocols and encouraging patient participation in rehabilitation efforts [30, 38, 39]. Malreduction causing loss of extension has been mentioned above. Arthrofibrosis is a rare but severe form of knee stiffness that can also occur after a tibial spine injury or operative fixation of these fractures. It is poorly understood but thought to be related to a genetic disposition for hypertrophic scar formation. Such aggressive inflammation causes intra-articular scar formation and loss of both flexion and extension. Patients within 3 months of surgery can be considered for postoperative joint manipulation to gain additional degrees of flexion.

Growth disruption in skeletally immature individuals is a potential complication, but with small drill holes and avoiding fixation across the physis, it is very uncommon [33, 45, 46].

2.10 Results and Outcomes

Tibial eminence fractures are relatively uncommon, and because of this, the literature and our knowledge about patient outcomes are limited. Most published case studies have low numbers and do not discriminate between adult and pediatric patients. A patient's outcome after tibial eminence fracture depends on many factors: degree of initial injury, operative versus nonoperative management, timing of treatment, type of fixation, rehabilitation protocols, and patient compliance.

Most patients do well after tibial eminence fractures if they are treated appropriately. Overall, the literature demonstrates significantly less laxity and loss of range of motion in patients with type I and II fractures than those with completely displaced fractures. As previously mentioned, nonoperative management has a role in the treatment of nondisplaced or minimally displaced fractures. Good results have been reported with regard to range of motion, stability, bony union, residual pain, and return to sport in these situations [13]. Subjective measures such as the IKDC scores, Lysholm scores, and Tegner scores are generally favorable [15, 26]. It appears that objective outcomes are improved with early motion and mobilization after treatment [28, 39, 40].

Several papers have reported poor results for type III fractures treated nonoperatively [47–49]. A retrospective case study of 61 pediatric patients found a direct correlation between fracture displacement and knee laxity [26]. Thus, most displaced fractures undergo arthroscopic reduction internal fixation (ARIF) or open reduction internal fixation (ORIF). A recent meta-analysis reviewed a total of 308 knees from 16 different studies and demonstrates the superiority of operative fixation in displaced tibial eminence fractures. Even though return to sport was similar between the nonoperative and operative groups, pooled analysis of displaced tibial eminence fractures revealed that nonoperatively treated patients more often report subjective instability. Additionally, this study revealed that 70 % of patients treated nonoperatively experience poor objective outcomes (KT-1000, Lachman, etc.), in stark comparison to the 14 % of patients who underwent surgical intervention. ACL reconstruction was ten times more common in the non-operatively treated patients [4].

With regard to the method of operative fixation, there is insufficient evidence to conclude the superiority of open versus arthroscopic fixation [50]. Watts et al. retrospectively reviewed patients under 18 years and found that an open approach was not an independent risk factor of arthrofibrosis [51]. No comment on the standard of care can be made, as both ORIF and ARIF are acceptable treatments for displaced tibial eminence fractures. However, arthroscopic techniques are growing in popularity and less invasive techniques are generally preferred.

When comparing suture and screw fixation, both methods appeared effective in restoring a patient's subjective feeling of knee stability. It is recommended that comminuted type IV fractures be treated with suture fixation, as bone stock is usually inadequate to achieve satisfactory screw purchase. As previously mentioned, biomechanical studies have not supported a clearly superior technique of fixation [34–37]. Seon et al. compared suture and screw fixation in type II and III fractures without functional differences [52]. Additionally, the incidence of subsequent ACL reconstruction is similar between the two methods of fixation [4]. Repeat surgery for hardware removal has been shown to have a higher incidence in patients treated with screw fixation, with 65 % of patients electing to undergo additional procedures [4].

As previously mentioned, very few patients struggle with nonunion or delayed unions regardless of treatment but are most common in displaced fractures treated with casting. There are few case reports in the literature describing ACL reconstruction, revision debridement, or fixation for the symptomatic patient with a nonunion or delayed union [40–42]. In nonunion or delayed union fractures of the anterior tibial spine, screw fixation is recommended over suture fixation [43]. Malunions can occur if reduction is unacceptable or if initial fixation is inadequate. These are rare but may result in flexion contractures requiring revision surgery [53]. There are very few reported cases of late complications such as growth arrest or hardware failure in the literature. Physeal-sparing techniques decrease the risk of growth arrest and ensuring adequate fixation intraoperatively will keep these complications to a minimum, ultimately improving patient outcomes.

References

1. Poncet A (1875) Arrachement de l'epine du tibia a l'insertion du ligament croise anterieur. Bull Mem Soc Chir Paris 1:883–884
2. Skak SV, Jensen TT, Poulsen TD, Sturup J (1987) Epidemiology of knee injuries in children. Acta Orthop Scand 58:78–81
3. Anderson CN, Anderson AF (2011) Tibial eminence fractures. Clin Sports Med 30:727–742
4. Bogunovic L, Tarabichi M, Harris D, Wright R (2015) Treatment of tibial eminence fractures: a systematic review. J Knee Surg 28:255–262
5. Lubowitz JH, Elson WS, Guttmann D (2005) Part II: arthroscopic treatment of tibial plateau fractures: intercondylar eminence avulsion fractures. Arthrosc J Arthrosc Relat Surg Off Publ Arthrosc Assoc N Am Int Arthrosc Assoc 21:86–92
6. Luhmann SJ (2003) Acute traumatic knee effusions in children and adolescents. J Pediatr Orthop 23:199–202
7. Eiskjaer S, Larsen ST, Schmidt MB (1988) The significance of hemarthrosis of the knee in children. Arch Orthop Trauma Surg 107:96–98
8. Kogan MG, Marks P, Amendola A (1997) Technique for arthroscopic suture fixation of displaced tibial intercondylar eminence fractures. Arthrosc J Arthrosc Relat Surg Off Publ Arthrosc Assoc N Am Int Arthrosc Assoc 13:301–306
9. Kocher MS, Micheli LJ, Gerbino P, Hresko MT (2003) Tibial eminence fractures in children: prevalence of meniscal entrapment. Am J Sports Med 31:404–407
10. Lafrance RM, Giordano B, Goldblatt J, Voloshin I, Maloney M (2010) Pediatric tibial eminence fractures: evaluation and management. J Am Acad Orthop Surg 18:395–405
11. Meyers MH, Mc KF (1959) Fracture of the intercondylar eminence of the tibia. J Bone Joint Surg Am 41-A:209–220; discussion 20–22
12. Aderinto J, Walmsley P, Keating JF (2008) Fractures of the tibial spine: epidemiology and outcome. Knee 15:164–167
13. Wilfinger C, Castellani C, Raith J, Pilhatsch A, Hollwarth ME, Weinberg AM (2009) Nonoperative treatment of tibial spine fractures in children-38 patients with a minimum follow-up of 1 year. J Orthop Trauma 23:519–524
14. Casalonga A, Bourelle S, Chalencon F, De Oliviera L, Gautheron V, Cottalorda J (2010) Tibial intercondylar eminence fractures in children: the long-term perspective. Orthop Traumatol Surg Research OTSR 96:525–530
15. Wiley JJ, Baxter MP (1990) Tibial spine fractures in children. Clin Orthop Relat Res 54–60
16. Kocher MS, Foreman ES, Micheli LJ (2003) Laxity and functional outcome after arthroscopic reduction and internal fixation of displaced tibial spine fractures in children. Arthrosc J Arthrosc Relat Surg Off Publ Arthrosc Assoc N Am Int Arthrosc Assoc 19:1085–1090
17. Noyes FR, DeLucas JL, Torvik PJ (1974) Biomechanics of anterior cruciate ligament failure: an analysis of strain-rate sensitivity and mechanisms of failure in primates. J Bone Joint Surg Am 56:236–253
18. Griffith JF, Antonio GE, Tong CW, Ming CK (2004) Cruciate ligament avulsion fractures. Arthrosc J Arthrosc Relat Surg Off Publ Arthrosc Assoc N Am Int Arthrosc Assoc 20:803–812
19. Zaricznyj B (1977) Avulsion fracture of the tibial eminence: treatment by open reduction and pinning. J Bone Joint Surg Am 59:1111–1114
20. Beaty JH, Kumar A (1994) Fractures about the knee in children. J Bone Joint Surg Am 76:1870–1880
21. Willis RB, Blokker C, Stoll TM, Paterson DC, Galpin RD (1993) Long-term follow-up of anterior tibial eminence fractures. J Pediatr Orthop 13:361–364
22. Fyfe IS, Jackson JP (1981) Tibial intercondylar fractures in children: a review of the classification and the treatment of mal-union. Injury 13:165–169
23. Mulhall KJ, Dowdall J, Grannell M, McCabe JP (1999) Tibial spine fractures: an analysis of outcome in surgically treated type III injuries. Injury 30:289–292
24. Molander ML, Wallin G, Wikstad I (1981) Fracture of the intercondylar eminence of the tibia: a review of 35 patients. J Bone Joint Surg 63-B:89–91
25. McLennan JG (1982) The role of arthroscopic surgery in the treatment of fractures of the intercondylar eminence of the tibia. J Bone Joint Surg 64:477–480
26. Janarv PM, Westblad P, Johansson C, Hirsch G (1995) Long-term follow-up of anterior tibial spine fractures in children. J Pediatr Orthop 15:63–68
27. Matthews DE, Geissler WB (1994) Arthroscopic suture fixation of displaced tibial eminence fractures. Arthrosc J Arthrosc Relat Surg Off Publ Arthrosc Assoc N Am Int Arthrosc Assoc 10:418–423
28. Berg EE (1993) Comminuted tibial eminence anterior cruciate ligament avulsion fractures: failure of arthroscopic treatment. Arthrosc J Arthrosc Relat Surg Off Publ Arthrosc Assoc N Am Int Arthrosc Assoc 9:446–450

29. Hunter RE, Willis JA (2004) Arthroscopic fixation of avulsion fractures of the tibial eminence: technique and outcome. Arthrosc J Arthrosc Relat Surg Off Publ Arthrosc Assoc N Am Int Arthrosc Assoc 20:113–121

30. Huang TW, Hsu KY, Cheng CY et al (2008) Arthroscopic suture fixation of tibial eminence avulsion fractures. Arthrosc J Arthrosc Relat Surg Off Publ Arthrosc Assoc N Am Int Arthrosc Assoc 24:1232–1238

31. Kim SJ, Shin SJ, Choi NH, Cho SK (2001) Arthroscopically assisted treatment of avulsion fractures of the posterior cruciate ligament from the tibia. J Bone Joint Surg Am 83-A:698–708

32. Lehman RA Jr, Murphy KP, Machen MS, Kuklo TR (2003) Modified arthroscopic suture fixation of a displaced tibial eminence fracture. Arthrosc J Arthrosc Relat Surg Off Publ Arthrosc Assoc N Am Int Arthrosc Assoc 19, E6

33. Hirschmann MT, Mayer RR, Kentsch A, Friederich NF (2009) Physeal sparing arthroscopic fixation of displaced tibial eminence fractures: a new surgical technique. Knee Surg Sports Traumatol Arthrosc Off J ESSKA 17:741–747

34. Bong MR, Romero A, Kubiak E et al (2005) Suture versus screw fixation of displaced tibial eminence fractures: a biomechanical comparison. Arthrosc J Arthrosc Relat Surg Off Publ Arthrosc Assoc N Am Int Arthrosc Assoc 21:1172–1176

35. Eggers AK, Becker C, Weimann A et al (2007) Biomechanical evaluation of different fixation methods for tibial eminence fractures. Am J Sports Med 35:404–410

36. Tsukada H, Ishibashi Y, Tsuda E, Hiraga Y, Toh S (2005) A biomechanical comparison of repair techniques for anterior cruciate ligament tibial avulsion fracture under cyclic loading. Arthrosc J Arthrosc Relat Surg Off Publ Arthrosc Assoc N Am Int Arthrosc Assoc 21:1197–1201

37. Mahar AT, Duncan D, Oka R, Lowry A, Gillingham B, Chambers H (2008) Biomechanical comparison of four different fixation techniques for pediatric tibial eminence avulsion fractures. J Pediatr Orthop 28:159–162

38. Vander Have KL, Ganley TJ, Kocher MS, Price CT, Herrera-Soto JA (2010) Arthrofibrosis after surgical fixation of tibial eminence fractures in children and adolescents. Am J Sports Med 38:298–301

39. Patel NM, Park MJ, Sampson NR, Ganley TJ (2012) Tibial eminence fractures in children: earlier posttreatment mobilization results in improved outcomes. J Pediatr Orthop 32:139–144

40. Kawate K, Fujisawa Y, Yajima H, Sugimoto K, Habata T, Takakura Y (2005) Seventeen-year follow-up of a reattachment of a nonunited anterior tibial spine avulsion fracture. Arthrosc J Arthrosc Relat Surg Off Publ Arthrosc Assoc N Am Int Arthrosc Assoc 21:760

41. Panni AS, Milano G, Tartarone M, Fabbriciani C (1998) Arthroscopic treatment of malunited and nonunited avulsion fractures of the anterior tibial spine. Arthrosc J Arthrosc Relat Surg Off Publ Arthrosc Assoc N Am Int Arthrosc Assoc 14:233–240

42. Horibe S, Shi K, Mitsuoka T, Hamada M, Matsumoto N, Toritsuka Y (2000) Nonunited avulsion fractures of the intercondylar eminence of the tibia. Arthrosc J Arthrosc Relat Surg Off Publ Arthrosc Assoc N Am Int Arthrosc Assoc 16:757–762

43. Vargas B, Lutz N, Dutoit M, Zambelli PY (2009) Nonunion after fracture of the anterior tibial spine: case report and review of the literature. J Pediatr Orthop B 18:90–92

44. Keys GW, Walters J (1988) Nonunion of intercondylar eminence fracture of the tibia. J Trauma 28:870–871

45. Vega JR, Irribarra LA, Baar AK, Iniguez M, Salgado M, Gana N (2008) Arthroscopic fixation of displaced tibial eminence fractures: a new growth plate-sparing method. Arthrosc J Arthrosc Relat Surg Off Publ Arthrosc Assoc N Am Int Arthrosc Assoc 24:1239–1243

46. Johnson DL, Durbin TC (2012) Physeal-sparing tibial eminence fracture fixation with a headless compression screw. Orthopedics 35:604–608

47. McLennan JG (1995) Lessons learned after second-look arthroscopy in type III fractures of the tibial spine. J Pediatr Orthop 15:59–62

48. Oostvogel HJ, Klasen HJ, Reddingius RE (1988) Fractures of the intercondylar eminence in children and adolescents. Arch Orthop Trauma Surg 107:242–247

49. Tudisco C, Giovarruscio R, Febo A, Savarese E, Bisicchia S (2010) Intercondylar eminence avulsion fracture in children: long-term follow-up of 14 cases at the end of skeletal growth. J Pediatr Orthop B 19:403–408

50. Gans I, Baldwin KD, Ganley TJ (2013) Treatment and management outcomes of tibial eminence fractures in pediatric patients: a systematic review. Am J Sports Med 42:1743–1750

51. Watts CD, Larson AN, Milbrandt TA (2015) Open versus arthroscopic reduction for tibial eminence fracture fixation in children. J Pediatr Orthop

52. Seon JK, Park SJ, Lee KB et al (2009) A clinical comparison of screw and suture fixation of anterior cruciate ligament tibial avulsion fractures. Am J Sports Med 37:2334–2339

53. Luger EJ, Arbel R, Eichenblat MS, Menachem A, Dekel S (1994) Femoral notchplasty in the treatment of malunited intercondylar eminence fractures of the tibia. Arthrosc J Arthrosc Relat Surg Off Publ Arthrosc Assoc N Am Int Arthrosc Assoc 10:550–551

Management of Distal Femoral Fractures (Extra-articular)

3

Seth R. Yarboro and Robert F. Ostrum

Abstract

Extra-articular distal femur fractures are challenging orthopedic injuries that occur less commonly than proximal and diaphyseal femur fractures. As implant design and technology improve, the rate of fracture healing and complication rate have both improved. Currently, these injuries are most commonly treated with lateral locking plates or intramedullary nail fixation, but have yet to show uniformly good results. Considerations to direct the appropriate implant choice include degree of comminution, distance above the joint line, and intra-articular extension. Complications of distal femur fixation include nonunion, implant failure, and malalignment. These complications may have severe impact on functional and radiographic outcomes, and strategies to achieve appropriate alignment and fixation of femur fractures must be carefully considered to achieve optimal results.

3.1 Epidemiology

Like many traumatic fractures, distal femur fractures occur in a bimodal distribution, with high-energy injuries seen in young patients and low-energy injuries in osteoporotic elderly patients. These fractures represent less than 1 % of all fractures and are less common than femoral shaft and proximal femur fractures, making up only about 5 % of femur fractures [1]. Five to ten percent of distal femur fractures have been reported to be open fractures [2], though other studies have demonstrated higher rates [2, 13].

3.2 Traumatic Mechanism

Mechanism of injury may involve axial loading, bending forces, rotation, or any combination therein. The fracture pattern may reflect the mechanism of injury (i.e., spiral fracture in setting of rotational injury or comminution in high-energy

S.R. Yarboro, MD (✉)
Department of Orthopaedics,
University of Virginia, 400 Ray C. Hunt Drive,
Suite 330, Charlottesville, VA 22903, USA
e-mail: seth.yarboro@gmail.com

R.F. Ostrum, MD
Department of Orthopaedics,
University of North Carolina, Chapel Hill, NC, USA

© Springer International Publishing Switzerland 2016
F. Castoldi, D.E. Bonasia (eds.), *Fractures Around the Knee*, Fracture Management Joint by Joint,
DOI 10.1007/978-3-319-28806-2_3

axial loading). High-energy mechanisms also result in a relatively large degree of soft tissue stripping from the bone and may ultimately result in open fractures. The open wounds associated with fractures are typically anterior and involve injury to the quadriceps tendon to a variable degree. The high-energy injuries are commonly reported to occur through motor vehicle or motorcycle crash, whereas the low-energy injuries often result from a fall from standing height.

3.3 Clinical Examination

Clinical exam begins with advanced trauma life support (ATLS) protocol, especially for higher-energy mechanism of injury. Limb-specific evaluation first involves the neurovascular exam to detail perfusion or nerve compromise. The skin must also be inspected for evidence of open fracture. The resting position of the lower extremity is examined for gross deformity, and the hip, thigh, and knee are evaluated for instability. Swelling and bruising are often seen at the level of injury. Compartment syndrome must be considered and ruled out at the time of initial exam. Ligamentous examination of the knee may be difficult due to proximity of the femur fracture, but should be considered.

3.4 Imaging and Preoperative Workup

Plain radiographs with orthogonal views of the entire length of the femur must be obtained to fully evaluate the distal femur fracture and to rule out ipsilateral femur fractures at other levels. The distance from the joint is measured, as this is important when considering implant choice.

CT scan is helpful to evaluate comminution, intercondylar extension (covered in the intra-articular distal femur chapter), and coronal plane fractures (Hoffa fracture).

Any concern for vascular injury would be an indication to obtain an ankle-brachial index (ABI). Any patient with a suspected vascular injury and ABI less than 0.9 should be evaluated by vascular surgery and have lower extremity angiography performed.

3.5 Classification

For practical purposes, many orthopedists use a descriptive classification of distal femur fracture patterns. However, the AO/OTA classification is the most commonly applied to the distal femur. AO/OTA classification for extra-articular distal femur fractures is denoted 33A. The extra-articular fractures are further divided into 33A-1, 33A-2, and 33A-3, indicating simple, metaphyseal wedge, or comminuted fracture pattern, respectively (Fig. 3.1). 33B and 33C (partial articular and complete articular, respectively) fractures will be covered in a separate chapter.

3.6 Indications

Most fractures of the distal femur require reduction and stable internal fixation to restore alignment and allow early range of motion. Nonoperative management is typically only appropriate for stable, nondisplaced fractures, or it is reserved for those patients who are nonambulatory or too medically unstable to tolerate surgery.

Fractures of the femoral shaft distal to the midshaft of the bone (infraisthmal) are good indications for an intramedullary (IM) nail. Extra-articular distal femur (supracondylar) fractures are amenable to a retrograde nail as well, but the surgeon must be sure that at least two screws, preferably out of plane to each other, can be inserted into the distal fracture segment. A simple coronal split in the articular cartilage can be fixed with a cancellous screw, and then a retrograde IM nail can be inserted as long as careful pre-op planning assures that the implants will not interfere with each other. Coronal fractures of the condyles can easily be managed with screw fixation remote from the IM nail insertion site and can be done before or after the IM nail procedure. With the increased incidence of both total knee replacements and osteoporosis, retrograde IM nailing of periprosthetic fractures can lead to a stable construct that may even allow some partial weight bearing due to the load-sharing properties of the IM nail. With all very distal femur fractures, it is incumbent upon the surgeon to examine the x-rays for intra-articular fracture lines and also to deter-

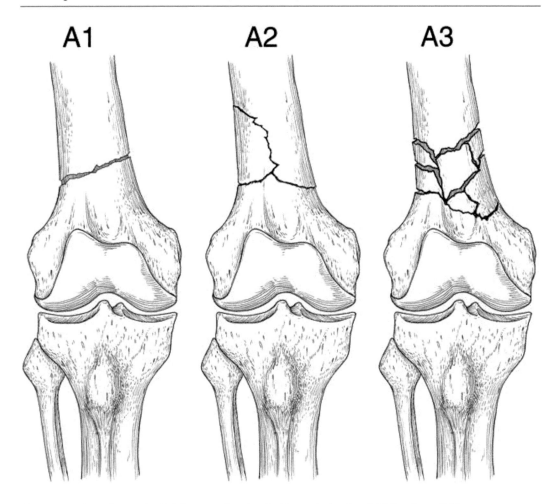

Fig. 3.1 AO/OTA diagram for 33A fractures (Reprinted with permission from FW Gwathmey [16])

mine the total amount of distal femur available for screw fixation. Remembering that the IM nail will be inserted just proximal to the intercondylar notch and knowing the location of the screw holes in the IM nail for distal interlocking will allow the surgeon to stabilize distal fractures with an IM nail when these parameters are met.

When a fracture is too distal to allow adequate fixation with the distal interlock screws of an IM nail, a lateral distal femur locking plate may provide a better option. The plate can be positioned quite distally if needed, with multiple screws available for fixation at the level of the condyles and metaphysis. Newer, variable angle locking plates are also now available that may provide the surgeon with improved ability to stabilize a wider range of fracture patterns.

3.7   Surgical Techniques (Anesthesia, Patient Positioning, Surgical Approaches, Reduction, and Fixation Techniques)

3.7.1   Anesthesia

For any patient requiring surgical stabilization of a distal femur fracture, clearance or optimization for surgery by the primary medicine or trauma service is obtained. Thorough evaluation by the anesthesia team should also be undertaken, and general anesthesia is routinely used for the procedure. If the surgeon believes that the reduction might be difficult or that gaining length may be a challenge, then it is incumbent for the surgeon to discuss the matter with the anesthesiologist and recommend general endotracheal anesthesia with complete muscle paralysis. In cases where the surgeon does not require paralysis, an effective spinal or epidural block may work as well, and these techniques have the added benefit of postoperative pain control. Regional anesthesia with a femoral nerve block may be a useful adjunct.

3.7.2 Patient Positioning

For all procedures, patients are placed in the supine position, with consideration of a blanket bump under the ipsilateral hip to neutralize lower extremity rotation.

For retrograde IM nailing of distal femur fractures, the patient is placed supine on a radiolucent table with the knee placed over a radiolucent sterile triangle. The use of a bolster under the ipsilateral buttocks is optional; however, if the surgeon uses a bump, then care must be taken to assess rotation of the femur. If no bolster is used, the patella can typically be placed straight anterior to allow for proper rational alignment of the limb. The leg is then prepped and draped in the usual sterile fashion making sure that the drapes go up to the pelvis to allow room for proximal screw insertion, anterior to posterior, for a full-length IM nail.

Prior to the surgery, the alignment and reduction of the limb can be assessed under fluoroscopic guidance, and by moving the triangle and a roll of towels posterior to the distal femur and applying traction, an acceptable reduction prior can be obtained (Fig. 3.2a).

3.7.3 External Fixation

External fixation is used as a temporizing measure when definitive fixation is not appropriate, such as in the setting of severe soft tissue injury or damage control orthopedics (DCO) scenario.

Two 5.0-mm Schanz pins are placed in the femur shaft (proximal to the intended proximal extent of the definitive fixation if a plate will be used). The authors' preferred technique is to predrill with a 3.5-mm drill. In the tibia, two Schanz pins are placed using the same technique. 175-mm half-pins and 150-mm half-pins typically work well in the femur and tibia, respectively, for most nonobese patients. Longer pins may be required for very obese patients.

The knee may then be stabilized with a spanning construct consisting of either pin banks placed at the pins and a "diamond" frame with bars and connectors between pin banks or pin-to-bar connectors used to place multiple bars directly between proximal and distal pins (Fig. 3.3). Applying longitudinal traction while maintaining appropriate alignment of the limb will typically bring the fracture into acceptable alignment for tightening the external fixation construct. The knee is typically placed at 15–20° of flexion, though this may be adjusted to accommodate fracture characteristics.

3.7.4 Intramedullary Devices

For the majority of extra-articular fractures, a small medial parapatellar tendon incision from the inferior pole of the patella to the tibial tubercle with either a medial or patellar tendon splitting incision will be sufficient to gain access to the insertion site. The knee on the triangle should be flexed between 30° and 45° to allow for passage of the reamers and IM nail. Too much flexion can bring the patella inferior and block the insertion site and too little flexion could possibly damage the tibial plateau. The synovium is spread, and a guide pin inserted into the distal femur and centered on both the AP and lateral fluoroscopic views. On the lateral view, with both femoral condyles superimposed on each other, the starting point should be 6 mm proximal to the convergence of Blumensaat's line and the femoral groove [3] (Fig. 3.2b, c). The AP view should show the pin centered in the distal femur, not perpendicular to the articular surface. A starting rigid reamer can be used over the guide pin while protecting the tendon and surrounding cartilage.

A ball-tipped long guide rod is then inserted across the fracture site up to the level at or above

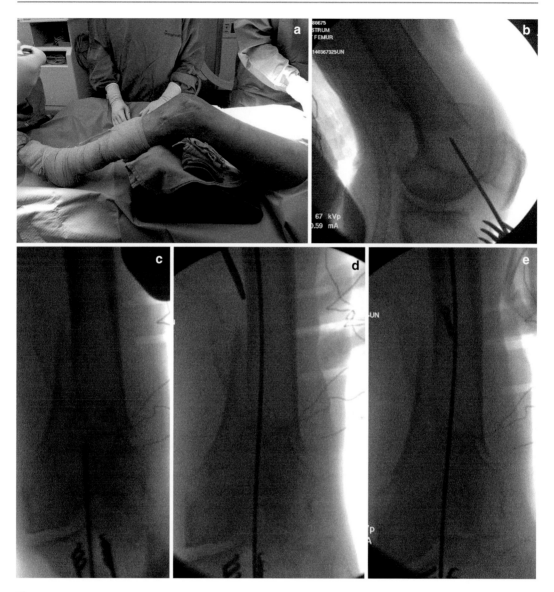

Fig. 3.2 (a) Lateral view showing distal femur fracture positioning over radiolucent triangle with bolsters behind the distal femur to correct apex posterior angulation. (b, c) A 90-year-old male with asymptomatic arthritis of the knee and supracondylar femur fracture. (b) Shows proper placement for retrograde IM nail on the lateral view just a few millimeters proximal to Blumensaat's line. (c) Shows anterior-posterior fluoroscopic view with guide pin centered in the distal femoral metaphysis. (d, e) – d Demonstrates medial translation of the distal femur after guide rod insertion. Note the guide rod centered in the distal femur but hugging the medial cortex at the infraisthmal femoral flare. (e) A blocking screw has been placed to block the IM nail from going along the medial cortex of the femur and thereby translating the distal femur laterally. (f, g) Final anterior-posterior x-rays showing excellent final alignment without translation or angulation of the distal femur. Due to the patient's age and osteoporosis, multiple screws with minimal purchase were used off-axis for distal femoral fixation. (g) Shows lateral radiograph and alignment. The blocking screw backed up slightly on IM nail insertion but is doing its job and should not be removed after IM nail insertion. The retrograde IM nail is not prominent at the level of the cartilage of the knee, and the alignment is satisfactory

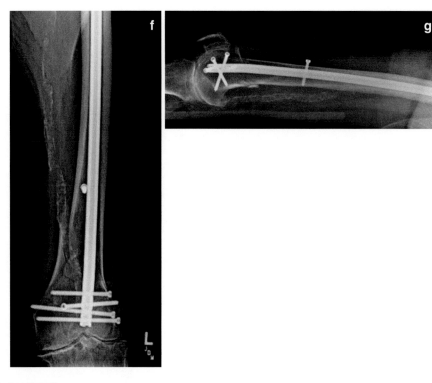

Fig. 3.2 (continued)

the lesser trochanter. For supracondylar fractures, it is imperative to maintain reduction while inserting the guide rod and during reaming. Reaming the intramedullary canal with the femoral fracture reduced will lead to better alignment once the IM nail is inserted, as it will not follow an aberrant track. The nail length is then determined using a ruler, and the proximal tip of the IM nail should be above the bottom of the lesser trochanter. Reaming is performed assuring that the reduction is maintained during this process. The intramedullary canal is reamed to 1 mm to 1.5 mm greater than the canal diameter that has been determined by the first reamer that contacted the cortex and caused audible "chatter." The retrograde IM nail is then inserted with the fracture reduction maintained. Close attention should be paid when the IM nail is crossing the fracture site as an eccentric entry into the proximal fragment can cause comminution. Using anterior-posterior and lateral fluoroscopy, visualization of the proximal end (insertion end) of the IM nail must be identified and its relationship to the intercondylar notch is

imperative. The nail must be at least flushed with the articular cartilage or even inserted deep to the cartilage by a few millimeters; it cannot be prominent as that will cause damage to the cartilage of the patella [4].

Distal interlocking is performed with an outrigger jig attached to the insertion handle of the IM nail. One screw is probably sufficient for stable, transverse fractures with greater than 50 % cortical contact. Two screws may be used when there is cortical comminution at the fracture site and oblique screws should be considered with small distal fragments in an attempt to get orthogonal screw placement. After distal interlocking, the length of the femur must be assessed. If the fracture does not have axial stability, the leg will shorten with IM nail insertion. When shortening is identified, following distal interlocking, the IM nail is "backslapped" to regain length and the fracture alignment is reassessed by fluoroscopy.

The insertion handle can then be removed and the leg can be placed flat on the OR table. If no bolster under the torso was used (author's

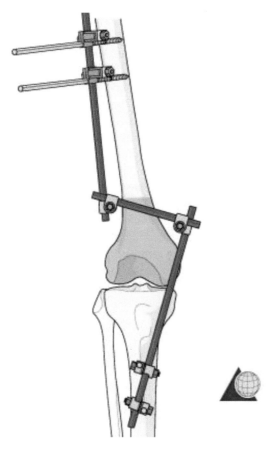

Fig. 3.3 "Z" configuration for knee spanning external fixator. Note that this construct does not require pin banks and can be planned to allow access to the distal femur so that it may remain in place at the time of definitive internal fixation (Reprinted with permission from AO Trauma)

preference), then the patella can be placed in a straight anterior direction during nail insertion and for proximal interlocking. The anterior to posterior proximal interlocking screws are placed using a "free-hand" technique and "perfect circles." The C-arm is positioned in an anterior to posterior position and an image of the proximal locking screws is obtained. The direction of the fluoroscopic image is changed until the anterior and posterior holes in the IM nail are collinear and appear as a "perfect circle." A small anterior incision is made over the proximal screw hole through the skin, quadriceps fascia, and the muscle down to the anterior cortex. The bayonet tip drill bit is then laid on the anterior cortex obliquely until the tip of the drill point is centered

in the proximal interlocking hole. The surgeon's arm is then brought to a position parallel to the direction of the C-arm, and the drill is inserted through the anterior cortex. Most commonly after this, the drill bit remains in the cortex but the drill is removed from the bit. The fluoroscopic view will determine the exact position that the drill bit has to go to make its way through the hole, and adjustments on the drill bit and its tip with gentle mallet blows can assist in getting the drill through the interlocking hole. The posterior cortex is drilled being careful not to over penetrate the posterior cortex and possibly injure the sciatic nerve. Utilizing a locking screwdriver, the screw is inserted after measuring with a depth gauge. Two proximal screws may be used for comminuted fractures. A full-length IM nail extending proximal to the bottom of the lesser trochanter should be used to prevent coronal plane motion and stress at the proximal end of the IM nail.

For supracondylar fractures, occasionally the alignment of the distal femur is not acceptable despite all of the "tricks" used for reduction, reaming, and insertion. In these cases, a blocking screw can be used to guide the IM nail into the desired position. Oftentimes, the IM nail must be removed, the long guidewire replaced into the femur, and using the short drill bit for the proximal interlocking screws, a hole is drilled next to the guide rod on the concave side of the deformity (Fig. 3.2d, e). The screw must block the IM nail's trajectory but allow enough room for the IM nail to pass. The screws utilized are those employed for interlocking the IM nail [5]. The retrograde nail is then reinserted and should "bounce" off of the blocking screw for this technique to work (Fig. 3.2f, g). Sometimes, the limb deformity must be exaggerated to allow the nail to proceed past the blocking screw. Proximal and distal interlocking is then performed as previously discussed, and the blocking screw is left in place to maintain the reduction.

After a layered closure, the leg is wrapped with a long elastic bandage from toes to groin. Immediate knee range of motion is stressed early in the rehabilitation process. Active motion is encouraged in cooperative, alert patients, and continuous passive motion (CPM) machines can be used for patients who are intubated or unable to comply with the therapy regimen. Transverse fractures with greater than 50 % cortical contact can start some immediate weight bearing and progress to full weight bearing as tolerated. Those patients with comminuted, length unstable fractures should start early partial weight bearing but refrain from full weight bearing until callus is visible on x-ray. By 6 weeks following surgery, most patients will have at least 90° of knee flexion, and by 3 months all patients should have near normal flexion.

3.7.5 Plate Fixation

Open reduction internal fixation with anatomically precontoured lateral plate is perhaps the current gold standard for distal femur fixation. Distal femur fractures involving the articular surface are addressed in a separate chapter.

The approach for distal femur plating will depend on the fracture pattern and exposure required to adequately address the injury. Minimally invasive plate osteosynthesis (MIPO) incisions are appropriate for simple fracture patterns or extra-articular patterns amenable to indirect reduction and bridge plating. However, this approach can be extended into a longer lateral incision for more extensive fractures that require direct reduction. Lastly, those fractures with intra-articular involvement that require access to the anterior distal femur may be approached through a lateral parapatellar arthrotomy that extends proximally to the lateral femur (termed "swashbuckler" approach). This approach is covered in the intra-articular distal femur chapter.

For lateral exposure, direct reduction, and plate application, a lateral incision is marked out from the lateral epicondyle and extended proximally in line with the femoral shaft. The incision may be extended further distally if required to allow mobilization of the skin without excessive tension. Skin incision is made with a #10 blade and carried down to the IT band. IT band is divided in line with its fibers, and the

vastus lateralis is visualized. The vastus lateralis is retracted anteriorly and elevated from the lateral intermuscular septum. Perforating vessels are encountered proximally and hemostasis achieved with electrocautery. The dissection is carried distally to expose the distal lateral femur (at this point the dissection can be adjusted more anterior to include lateral arthrotomy if intra-articular exposure is required).

If a direct reduction is undertaken, the fracture site is debrided of interposed fragments for simple fracture patterns where absolute stability can be achieved. For comminuted fractures where bridge plating is most appropriate, the fracture site is not routinely debrided.

With paralysis in place, length can usually be achieved with manual traction. If achieving adequate length proves challenging, a femoral distractor may be used to achieve length. A bump is placed under the femur at the level of the fracture functions to relax the deforming pull of the gastrocnemius on the distal fragment and maintain the alignment of the shaft and metaphysis once achieved. For simple fracture patterns, periarticular reduction clamps (such as "King Tong" clamp) may assist with reduction and can be applied safely to the medial side of the femur with a small percutaneous stab incision or a folded OR towel to avoid injury to the skin [19]. Provisional fixation is then achieved with Kirschner wires.

Plate application is performed by sliding the plate under the vastus lateralis along the femoral shaft. Plate length can be determined by preoperative templating or by estimation during surgery followed by fluoroscopic confirmation of appropriate length. We recommend a minimum of four bicortical screws above the fracture site, taking into consideration adequate working length for bridge plate applications – typically a minimum of three empty holes remain at the level of the fracture for bridge plating, though this number may be greater for extensive comminution.

Stepwise, once appropriate plate length is established:

1. Provisional fixation of the plate at the distal femur using a k-wire, based on perfect lateral view (Fig. 3.4).

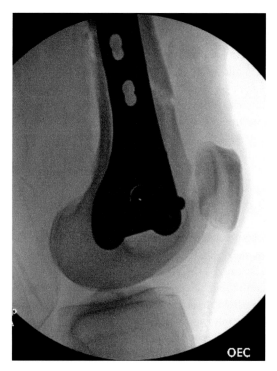

Fig. 3.4 Lateral view of the distal femur with appropriate plate position. Note that the distal/posterior most screw is posterior to Blumensaat's line, and a unicondylar screw was used in this position

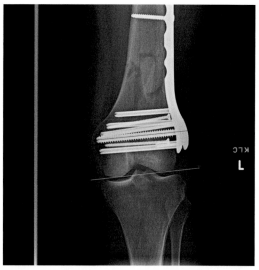

Fig. 3.5 Anatomically precontoured lateral locking plates are designed to recreate the normal valgus angle of the distal femur and should be placed parallel to the distal articular surface

2. Provisional fixation of the plate proximally with a k-wire. The plate should be centered on the shaft in the lateral view. This step avoids unrecognized plate malposition on the shaft.
3. On AP view, confirmation of appropriate varus/valgus alignment. Guidewire for first distal locking screw should be aligned with distal articular surface (Fig. 3.5).
4. Secure the shaft with 4.5-mm cortical screw.
5. Correct any remaining extension deformities of distal fragment with direct reduction prior to placing subsequent distal locking screws.
6. Place remaining shaft screws.

In the setting of severe bone loss or defect, Masquelet technique may be used. This technique is a two-stage strategy for the reconstruction of long bone segmental diaphyseal defects and utilizes induced membranes with nonvascularized bone autograft [17, 18]. The first stage involves placement of a polymethyl methacrylate (PMMA) cement spacer into the defect, with closure or soft tissue coverage of the area. Approximately 6 weeks later, the second stage consists of spacer removal with care taken to not disrupt the membrane around the defect. This cavity is filled with cancellous autograft bone that can be combined with demineralized bone matrix or allograft if additional volume is required. The technique relies on the theory that the biological membrane induced by the PMMA cement has a protective and positive effect on the cancellous autograft.

3.7.5.1 Tips

If shortening is accepted to improve bony apposition and excessive medial translation of the distal fragment is encountered, one may apply cortical screws in the proximal portion of the shaft, followed by locking screws for distal fixation of the shaft, which will appropriately secure the position of the distal fragment in the coronal plane (Fig. 3.6). This will avoid excessive medial translation of the condyle portion of the fracture.

For osteoporotic bone or very distal fractures, a more distal plate position may be chosen. The most distal posterior locking screw may still be

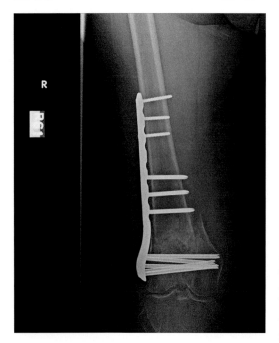

Fig. 3.6 This fracture demonstrated severe comminution, and shortening was accepted to improve contact at the fracture site. Locking screws in the distal portion of the shaft are an effective way to control its position, avoiding excessive medialization of the condylar fragment

placed across both condyles, accepting that the screw is intra-articular in the femoral notch (evaluated on the notch view of the knee). To avoid this scenario with a distal plate position, use a shorter screw that only traverses the lateral condyle.

3.8   Postoperative Regimen

Following placement of external fixator, patients are non-weight bearing until the time of definitive internal fixation. Low molecular weight heparin (LMWH) or other chemoprophylaxis is typically used for deep vein thrombosis (DVT) prophylaxis because of the considerable immobilization. Routine pin care is performed.

After plate fixation, patients are typically toe touch weight bearing (TTWB) for 6–8 weeks, using a walker or crutches to mobilize. DVT prophylaxis at our institution consists of 2 weeks of LMWH 40 mg subcutaneous (SC) daily, then four additional weeks of 325 mg aspirin (ASA)

by mouth daily. Antibiotics are continued postoperatively for two additional doses not to exceed 24 h after surgery.

Following IM nail fixation, activity level varies depending on factors including bone quality, amount of fixation, and degree of comminution, though earlier motion may be considered based on the load-sharing properties of the IM nail.

3.8.1   Rehabilitation

Immediate knee range of motion is stressed early in the rehabilitation process. Active motion is encouraged in cooperative, alert patients, and continuous passive motion (CPM) machines can be used for patients who are intubated or unable to comply with the therapy regimen. Since these fractures are infraisthmal, there is no good cortical contact, and for the majority of patients, limited initial weight bearing is usually recommended. Those patients with comminuted, length unstable fractures should start early partial weight bearing but refrain from full weight bearing until callus is visible on x-ray. By 6 weeks following surgery, most patients will have at least 90° of knee flexion, and by 3 months all patients should have near normal flexion.

3.9   Complications

1. *Coronal plane malalignment* – Anatomically precontoured lateral locking plates are designed to recreate the normal valgus angle of the distal femur, and certain implant-specific screws should be placed parallel to the distal articular surface (Fig. 3.5). Coronal plane malalignment will result in excessive loading of the medial or lateral compartment of the knee.

    With retrograde IM nailing of distal femur fractures, malalignment and malunion are possible due to the fact that there is no cortex to guide the nail. Varus and valgus are both possible and often the concavity of the deformity is on the more comminuted side. Blocking screws do act as an artificial cortex and can guide the IM nail into position, reduce the fracture, and decrease the incidence of malalignment.

2. *Incorrect implant position* – Placing the plate too anterior or posterior may result in intra-articular screws that violate the trochlea or notch, respectively. The distal femur has a trapezoidal shape, which must be considered to achieve safe implant placement. Posterior plate placement on the distal condylar fragment will lead to medial displacement or golf club deformity of the femur [14, 15]. Further, the proximal portion of the plate has a tendency to shift too anterior relative to the shaft. In this instance, the proximal locking screws may not engage the bone or only have unicortical purchase. This problem can be addressed by placing a percutaneous k-wire through the most proximal hole to maintain appropriate position during placement of the distal screws.

   Even for supracondylar fractures, a full-length retrograde femoral IM nail should be used to take advantage of the isthmus to prevent excessive movement of the implant in the femur. It is imperative with retrograde IM nailing to be absolutely sure that the distal tip of the IM nail is not prominent at the level of the articular cartilage.

3. *Prominent screws at medial cortex* – If distal screws are too long, they may encroach on the medial collateral ligament (MCL). This complication is likely to be symptomatic for patients and may require implant revision or removal. An internal rotation view along the medial aspect of the distal femur (approximately 25° rotated) will allow the surgeon to evaluate for prominent screws.

   The distal screws placed through the femoral condyles and through the IM nail can be symptomatic. A prominent screw head on the lateral condyle may be palpable and cause friction with knee motion as the iliotibial band rubs over it. Additionally, when the screws are a little too long, the medial tip of the screw often causes pain as it is prominent, and with knee flexion, the quadriceps rubs over the screw tip causing pain. Removal of screws is possible after 12 months when the fracture

appears to have remodeled callus surrounding the fracture site.

4. *Sagittal plane deformity* – The force of the gastrocnemius muscle on the distal fragment results in extension. This deformity should be anticipated, and knee flexion will decrease the deforming force and facilitate reduction. Patients may have excessive extension and gait abnormalities related to the malalignment. Apex anterior malalignment is perhaps less well tolerated compared to recurvatum deformity due to the inability to regain full knee extension.

5. *Nonunion* – Due to the metadiaphyseal location and the closed reduction of the distal femur fracture for IM nailing, the union rates are very high, greater than 90 %. The ability to perform the nailing procedure without disrupting the muscle or blood supply or disruption of the healing factors has led to few fractures that do not heal. If nonunion is present, then a workup can be performed to rule out systemic causes like Vitamin D deficiency or the use of blood thinners or steroids or other factor-inhibiting drugs. Similar results can be obtained with minimally invasive plating if the medial soft tissues are respected and left intact.

   One critical aspect of considering options for the treatment of nonunions is to assess the fracture stability. In an atrophic nonunion, if the hardware is stable, then a bone graft can be added. If the hardware is not stable, then either an exchange IM nail or plating can be performed with adjunctive bone grafting. For hypertrophic nonunion that just want more stability, an exchange IM nail or plating can be performed without the addition of bone graft.

6. *Decreased range of motion* – Knee stiffness following these fractures is not uncommon in those patients immobilized for a period of time following surgery or those who do not start early knee motion. The quadriceps scars down to the fracture and its effective working length is decreased. Further, if the patella is not mobilized, then there are intra-articular contractures as well. Early range of motion (ROM) and

physical therapy are the hallmarks of early aggressive treatment. Should this fail to regain motion after several months, then a knee manipulation in the operating room or a quadriceps-plasty may be required to regain knee flexion. Pillows behind the knee or prolonged sitting can lead to a flexion contracture of the knee, and patients are encouraged to get the knee to full extension while sitting or exercising.

7. *Infection* – Infection is rare following plating or retrograde IM nailing of distal femur fractures. Small nonhealing incisions can be treated expectantly with cleansing and possible antibiotics by mouth. If the knee joint shows evidence of infection following knee aspirate, then an arthrotomy is required to debride the synovium and active drain suction is recommended. Intravenous antibiotics may be necessary, and the IM nail or plate can be retained if the fracture has not healed yet and supplemented with suppressive antibiotic treatment. Hardware removal and local antibiotics may be employed as a definitive treatment once the surgeon is assured that the fracture is healed.

3.10   Results

Outcomes following fixation of distal femur fractures for both plate and IM nail fixation have been reported, and while modern implants have improved results compared to historical data, they have not resulted in uniformly good outcomes.

Early studies utilizing retrograde IM nails for distal femur fractures had good union rates, but malunions, shortening, painful and broken screws, as well as loss of reduction [6, 7]. Techniques improved as did the implants, and results with retrograde nails improved to be similar to those of plating. Three studies compared the results of plating versus retrograde I nailing of distal femur fractures. In 2004, Markmiller et al. found no difference in ROM in the less invasive stabilization system (LISS) plate versus retrograde groups and reported malunion in three plated femurs and two retrograde-nailed femurs [8]. At 1-year follow-up, nonunion and secondary surgical procedures were 10 % for both groups. A study comparing dynamic

condylar screw (DCS) to retrograde nailing for distal femur fractures in elderly patients revealed a shorter OR time with less blood loss in the IM nail group, but complications were equal as were union rates and clinical results [9]. Hartin et al. reported on 23 patients randomized to plate versus IM nail and found that three patients in the retrograde IM nail group required revision surgery and this group had more pain on the SF-36 outcome score [10].

Clinical results after retrograde IM nailing of periprosthetic fractures around total knee replacements have been good. Recently, Pelfort published that 7/30 patients treated with an IM nail after total knee replacement had a mean extension deformity of 18° but at 6 year follow-up had no clinical symptoms [11]. To consider retrograde IM nailing for periprosthetic fractures, the surgeon must know the design and specifications of the femoral component as well as the characteristics of the IM nail being employed. Heckler et al. reported on the size of the femoral components, and this reference can be helpful if the surgeon is considering IM nailing through a total knee replacement [12].

Hoffmann et al. evaluated outcomes following plate fixation of distal femur fractures in a retrospective cohort and found a 74.8 % union rate after the index procedure [13]. They did have an 18 % nonunion rate, and 20 % of those in the nonunion group went on to recalcitrant nonunion. Submuscular plating had a lower nonunion rate than open reduction (80.0 % healed versus 61.3 %). It should be noted that 40.5 % of the injuries in this series were open fractures. Gardner et al. in a series of 335 patients treated with locked plating reported an 81 % union rate after the primary procedure and a 5 % overall infection rate. Diabetes and open fracture were both independent risk factors for needing reoperation and for deep infection. Implant failure was associated with open fracture, smoking, higher BMI, and shorter plate length [2].

Conclusions
Extra-articular distal femur fractures continue to be challenging injuries. Although implants have become more versatile and tailored to

accommodate these specific fractures, care must be taken to avoid complications. Preoperative planning, implant selection, careful handling of soft tissue, restoration of alignment, and confirmation of appropriate implant position make up an important part of the approach required to maximize outcomes when treating this injury.

References

1. Martinet O, Cordey J, Harder Y et al (2000) The epidemiology of fractures of the distal femur. Injury 31(Suppl 3):C62–C63
2. Ricci WM, Streubel PN, Gardner MJ et al (2014) Risk factors for failure of locked plate fixation of distal femur fractures: an analysis of 335 cases. J Orthop Trauma 28:83–89
3. Carmack D, Moed B, Kingston C et al (2003) Identification of the optimal intercondylar starting point for retrograde femoral nailing: an anatomic study. J Trauma 55(4):692–695
4. Morgan E, Ostrum R, DiCicco J et al (1999) Effects of retrograde femoral intramedullary nailing on the patellofemoral articulation. J Orthop Trauma 13(1):13–16
5. Ostrum RF, Maurer JP (2009) Distal third femur fractures treated with retrograde femoral nailing and blocking screws. J Orthop Trauma 23(9):681–684
6. Lucas SE, Seligson D, Henry SL (1993) Intramedullary supracondylar nailing of femoral fractures. A preliminary report of the GSH supracondylar nail. Clin Orthop Relat Res 296:200–206
7. Handoiln L, Palarinen J, Lindahl J et al (2004) Retrograde intramedullary nailing in distal femoral fractures- results in a series of 46 consecutive operations. Injury 35(5):517–522
8. Markmiller M, Konrad G, Sudkamp N (2004) Femur-LISS and distal femoral nail for fixation of distal femoral fractures: are there differences in outcome and complications? Clin Orthop Relat Res 426: 252–257
9. Christodoulou A, Terzidis I, Ploumis A, Metsovitis S, Koukoulidis A, Toptsis C (2005) Supracondylar femoral fractures in elderly patients treated with the dynamic condylar screw and the retrograde intramedullary nail: a comparative study of the two methods. Arch Orthop Trauma Surg 125(2):73–79
10. Hartin NL, Harris I, Hazratwala K (2006) Retrograde nailing versus fixed-angle blade plating for supracondylar femoral fractures: a randomized control. ANZ J Surg 76(5):290–294
11. Pelfort X, Torres-Claramunt R, Hinarejos P et al (2013) Extension malunion of the femoral component after retrograde nailing: no sequelae at 6 years. J Orthop Trauma 27(3):158–161
12. Heckler MW, Tennant GS, Willaims P, DiCicco JD (2007) Retrograde nailing of supracondylar periprosthetic femur fractures: a surgeon's guide to femoral component sizing. Orthopaedics 30(5):345–350
13. Hoffmann MF, Jones CB, Koenig SJ et al (2013) Clinical outcomes of locked plating of distal femoral fractures in a retrospective cohort. J Orthop Surg Res 8:43
14. Beltran MJ, Gary JL, Collinge CA (2015) Management of distal femur fractures with modern plates and nails: state of the art. J Orthop Trauma 29(4):165–172
15. Collinge CA, Gardner MJ, Crist BD (2011) Pitfalls in the application of distal femur plates for fractures. J Orthop Trauma 25:695–706
16. Gwathmey FW, Jones-Quaidoo SM, Cui Q et al (2010) Distal femoral fractures: current concepts. J Am Acad Orthop Surg 18:597–607
17. Masquelet AC, Fitoussi F, Begue T et al (2000) Reconstruction of the long bones by the induced membrane and spongy autograft. Ann Chir Plast Esthet 45(3):346–353
18. Masquelet AC, Begue T (2010) The concept of induced membrane for reconstruction of long bone defects. Orthop Clin North Am 41(1):27–37
19. Alves K, Dahners LE (2012) A technical trick which reduces the need for stab incisions when using bone tenaculums for fracture reduction. J Orthop Trauma 26(6):e58–e59

Management of Distal Femoral Fractures (Intra-articular)

4

Mario Ronga, Giuseppe La Barbera,
Marco Valoroso, Giorgio Zappalà,
Jacopo Tamini, and Paolo Cherubino

Abstract

Isolated unicondylar distal femoral fractures are rare injuries. Most of them are associated to distal femoral fracture (55 %). The most common mechanism of injury is an axial load to the leg sometimes associated to varus, valgus, or rotation forces. After history and physical examination, X-rays and CT scan, including multiplanar and 3-D reconstructions, are mandatory. Several surgical exposures and different techniques and implants have been developed to achieve fracture healing, preserving the soft tissue, early knee motion, and functional recovery. The application of the principles of fixation for the different implants and the respect of indications are fundamental for a successful outcome.

4.1 Epidemiology

Distal femoral fractures, including supracondylar and intracondylar, represent less than 1 % of all fractures and about 3–6 % of all femoral fractures. They occur in a bimodal distribution: young male patients involved in high-energy trauma (traffic accident or a fall from heights) and elderly patients, in most cases female with poor bone quality, who sustain a low-energy trauma. Intra-articular involvement is present in 55 % of distal femoral fractures [10, 17].

Isolated unicondylar distal femoral fractures are rare injuries. Two different types of fracture can be observed: (1) the Hoffa fracture is defined as a coronally oriented fracture that more often involves the lateral condyle (less than ten cases have been reported in literature involving the medial condyle) [5, 44] and (2) the Trélat fracture that develops in sagittal plane affecting more frequently the medial condyle [5]. Unicondylar fractures commonly occur associated with complex intra-supracondylar femoral fractures. Hoffa fracture is present in approximately 40 % of intercondylar fractures, especially in open fractures (5–10 % of supracondylar fractures) [17, 44]. Associated ligament tears and meniscus

M. Ronga (✉) • G. La Barbera • M. Valoroso
G. Zappalà • J. Tamini • P. Cherubino
Orthopaedics and Traumatology, Department
of Biotechnology and Life Sciences (DBSV),
University of Insubria, Ospedale di Circolo,
Viale L. Borri 57, Varese 21100, Italy
e-mail: mario.ronga@uninsubria.it

© Springer International Publishing Switzerland 2016
F. Castoldi, D.E. Bonasia (eds.), *Fractures Around the Knee*, Fracture Management Joint by Joint,
DOI 10.1007/978-3-319-28806-2_4

lesions have been reported in approximately 20–70 % of cases [17]. Associated neurovascular injury is rarely reported. The femoral or popliteal artery lesion occurs in approximately 0.2 % of the cases, threatening the vitality of the whole limb, and therefore has to be carefully ruled out [25].

4.2   Traumatic Mechanism

The most common mechanism of injury is an axial load to the leg sometimes associated to varus, valgus, or rotation forces. In younger patients sustaining high-energy trauma, considerable fracture displacement, comminution, contamination, and associated injuries are present. In elderly with poor bone quality, fracture occurs during fall on a flexed knee [17, 25].

Unicondylar fracture occurs in high-velocity trauma. The proposed mechanism of injury consists of an axial load to the femoral condyle at 90° or more of knee flexion and results in a posterior tangential fracture pattern [5, 11, 44]. Fracture displacement is caused by the direction of the trauma and muscle contraction. Limb shortening and varus angulation depend on the contraction of the quadriceps, hamstrings, and adductor muscles. Posterior angulation of the apex and displacement of the distal fragment are caused by the contraction of the gastrocnemius. Rotational malalignment, in cases of intra-articular fracture, is caused by soft tissue attachments (capsule, ligaments, tendons) on the femoral condyles.

4.3   Clinical Examination

History and physical examination are fundamental to understand the fracture pattern and associated lesions. Patients complain of severe thigh or knee pain, with inability to weight bear on the affected side. Swelling, tenderness, fracture crepitans, and limb deformity (shortening and external rotation) are present at the clinical evaluation. The skin integrity has to be evaluated to identify possible open fractures. The most common open

fracture location is anterior, proximal to patella, through the quadriceps caused by penetration of spike fracture. A careful neurovascular evaluation of the affected extremity is fundamental before starting imaging studies [17, 25].

4.4   Imaging and Preoperative Workup

Anteroposterior (AP) and lateral (LL) radiographs are the first-line exams for evaluating the fracture. In high-energy trauma, X-rays of the pelvis, ipsilateral hip, and femoral shaft are recommended to recognize possible associated injuries. CT scan, including 3-D reconstruction, is recommended because the intra-articular involvement is present in 55 % of distal femoral fractures. Moreover, CT scan study is mandatory in complex intra-articular fractures to evaluate comminution degree and fracture lines in the coronal and sagittal planes [17].

Diagnosis of Hoffa fracture can be challenging and often requires clinical suspicion based on traumatic mechanism. X-rays are usually unremarkable. Nork et al. reported that Hoffa fractures are missed in 31 % of the cases with plain radiographies alone. In case of clinical suspicion, it is useful to obtain oblique radiographs that can help to define the fracture lines [30]. CT scan is helpful not only to identify the fracture but also to plan the treatment in terms of patient positioning, surgical approach, and fixation method [44].

4.5   Classification

Different distal femoral fracture classifications have been proposed in the literature [9, 37, 43]. The AO classification is the most used [29]. This system classifies extra-articular fracture as type A, partial articular/unicondylar fractures as type B, and complete articular/bicondylar fractures as type C. Every type is subclassified into three patterns according to the degree of comminution and instability [17, 25].

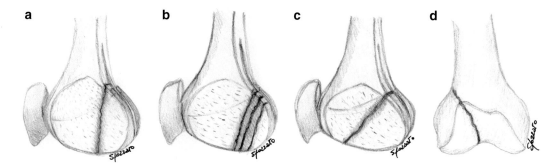

a   b   c   d

Fig. 4.1 Unicondylar fractures. (**a–c**). Classification of fractures of the femoral condyle according to Letenneur. (**a**). Type I is located in the posterior aspect of the femoral condyle being parallel to the posterior femoral cortex and extending from the femoral shaft-condylar junction to the posterior condylar articular surface. (**b**). Type II is a fracture originating posteriorly to the junction between femoral shaft and condyle, remaining parallel to the posterior femoral cortex. It may be intra-articular. Three subtypes are described according to the fragment size compared to type I: type A about 75 %, type B 50 %, type C 25 %. (**c**). Type III is an oblique fracture of the posterior aspect of the femoral condyle. (**d**). Trélat fracture develops in sagittal plane

Letenneur et al. classified Hoffa fractures into three types in order to predict which fractures would progress to avascular necrosis. However, no relationship between fracture type and avascular necrosis has been conclusively demonstrated. Fractures were classified into three types: type I is a fracture parallel to the posterior femoral cortex; type II occurs posterior to this line, but remains parallel to the posterior femoral cortex; and type III is an oblique fracture of the posterior femoral condyle (Fig. 4.1a–c). Soft tissue attachments (capsule, ligaments, tendons) are preserved in type I and III, while in type II are frequently not preserved [3, 24, 44]. Trélat fracture has been described as a unicondylar fracture developing in the sagittal plane [5] (Fig. 4.1d).

4.6   Indications

Intra-articular distal femoral fractures require surgical treatment due to better results compared to nonsurgical treatment in terms of union, alignment, range of motion, and functional outcome. Nonoperative treatment is indicated in cases of stable, nondisplaced fractures and when medical comorbidities contraindicate surgery (medical unsuitability, severe osteoporosis, and severe comminution) [17]. In a prospective, randomized controlled trial comparing surgical with nonsurgical management of displaced distal femoral fractures in elderly patients, Butt et al. observed higher rate of complications in the nonsurgical group, while better results were reported in the surgical group (53 % vs. 31 % respectively) [8].

Once the "personality" of the fracture has been defined, the surgeon can decide the appropriate surgical approach and fixation method. Fixed-angle side plates including blade plates, condylar plates with a sliding barrel, and locking plates can be used for intra-articular fractures and fractures in the osteoporotic bone. These plates may be indicated for the simple extra-articular (AO type A1) as well as the comminuted intra-articular (AO type C3) fractures. Buttress plates and screws can be used in relatively stable fracture and partial articular fractures (AO type B). They also can be implanted to augment other constructs. Intramedullary (IM) nailing is useful for extra-articular (AO type A) and in association with lag screws for simple or minimally comminuted intra-articular (AO types C1 and C2) fractures. External fixator is indicated as temporary treatment, applying the concept of the damage control: spanning external fixation to restore length and stabilize the extremity is used to allow patient systemic stabilization, especially in high-energy fractures with excessive soft tissue lesion and periosteal stripping as well as for open fractures with devitalized tissue and contamination.

Definitive internal fixation should be performed when the patient and soft tissue have improved. External fixation is indicated as definitive treatment in comminuted fractures, in severe open fractures, and in patients who are unsuitable for additional surgery. Total knee arthroplasty (TKA) is an option in select osteoporotic elderly patients with preexisting arthritis or severely comminuted fracture [17].

4.7 Surgical Techniques

The goal of surgery is to achieve anatomical reduction of the articular surface, correct axial alignment, and restoration of femoral length, regardless of the implant and the surgical technique. In the intra-articular fracture, restoration of the congruity of the articular surface should be a priority, and in complex fractures, the intercondylar part should be addressed before the metadiaphyseal part [7]. Length, alignment, and rotation should be evaluated clinically and fluoroscopically after reduction and before the implant fixation [3, 17, 44].

4.8 Patient Positioning

The patient is placed in supine position on a radiolucent table to allow adequate intraoperative fluoroscopic imaging of the whole lower limb. It is fundamental to evaluate preoperatively the contralateral limb to check the correct length, axes, and rotation. The operated thigh should be freely movable. The use of traction allows restoring the correct length of the femur. Traction can be manual, skeletal on proximal tibia, or with a universal distractor. Preparation and draping should allow complete exposure of the operated femur up to the hip joint. The knee should be flexed at 30° and the femur supported by paddings: this reduces the traction forces of the gastrocnemius muscle and prevents the extension of the distal fragment, reducing the recurvatum deformity and making the fracture reduction easier.

4.9 Surgical Approaches

Distal femoral approach depends on fracture pattern and implant used. The traditional open exposures are indicated in cases of intra-articular fracture comminution, while minimally invasive incisions are used to perform a bridge plating in case of simple articular/comminuted metaphyseal fracture or in retrograde nailing.

A lateral approach is indicated when plating fractures with simple undisplaced articular involvement (AO 33-C1). A curved lateral incision is made from Gerdy's tubercle and extended proximally, in-line with the femoral shaft (Fig. 4.2a). The lower margin of the vastus lateralis muscle is exposed. The iliotibial tract is split in the direction of its fibers, and the vastus lateralis muscle is reflected anteriorly to expose the distal femur. A lateral arthrotomy is then performed. This approach allows atraumatic elevation of the vastus lateralis muscle from the lateral aspect of the femur and a lateral arthrotomy for joint access. This approach allows an easy plate application, which is important to avoid malreduction and implant malpositioning. A swashbuckler approach is indicated for displaced articular fractures (AO 33-C2–33-C3), ensuring an optimal joint view (Fig. 4.2b, c) [7, 39].

In case of isolated medial femoral condyle fracture or in some cases of complex intra-articular fracture where a medial plate is required, a medial approach is required. The incision is centered over the fracture and extended to the adductor tubercle. The fascia is dived in-line with skin incision. Then the vastus medialis muscle is elevated to expose the distal femur. When articular exposure is needed, a medial parapatellar approach can be performed. It is necessary to dislocate laterally the patella to obtain a good view of the distal femur [17, 25]. However, Beltran et al. demonstrated that coronal fractures of the medial condyle can be adequately visualized using a mini-swashbuckler approach. Reduction and stabilization of the medial fragment can be achieved also through an accessory medial incision while working through a lateral approach [7].

In retrograde intramedullary nailing, the knee needs to be bent approximately at 70°. A 4 cm

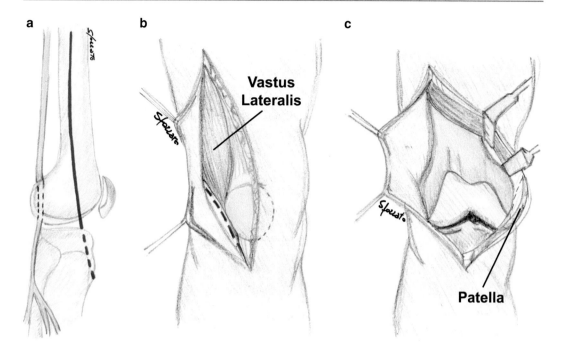

Fig. 4.2 Approaches to the distal femur. (**a**). *Lateral approach*. A curved lateral incision is made from Gerdy's tubercle and extended proximally, in-line with the femoral shaft (*red line*). The lower margin of the vastus lateralis muscle is exposed. The iliotibial tract is split in the direction of its fibers, and the vastus lateralis muscle is reflected anteriorly to expose the distal femur. After, a lateral arthrotomy is performed. The sciatic and common peroneal nerve (*yellow line*). (**b**). *Swashbuckler approach*. The incision is more anterior than the lateral approach. The joint is approached between the lateral patellar retinaculum and the vastus lateralis muscle and then through a lateral parapatellar arthrotomy (*dashed line*). (**c**). Quadriceps muscles and patella are reflected medially to expose the joint

midline skin incision is made, extending from the inferior pole of the patella to the tibial tubercle, followed by a medial parapatellar capsular incision. This should be sufficient to expose the intercondylar notch for retrograde nail insertion. The posterior cruciate ligament and the weight-bearing cartilage are the major structures to protect [7, 17, 25].

The approach to the Hoffa fractures is guided by the Letenneur classification. Lateral type I and III fractures can be managed by a lateral or swash-buckler approach. Lateral type II C fractures require a posterior approach, paying attention to popliteal vessels and nerves [44]. Agarwal et al. described a surgical approach to treat the rare bicondylar Hoffa fractures. These fractures require a tibial tubercle osteotomy to manage the reduction and fixation of the intra-articular fragments [1].

4.10   Simple Screw Fixation

Simple screw fixation is recommended in case of a frontal or sagittal unicondylar fracture. Usually the fracture is addressed through a medial or lateral parapatellar approach (Fig. 4.3). A percutaneous procedure is possible in case of minimal displacement when the reduction can be obtained with ligamentotaxis [13].

A recent study showed that osteosynthesis using two 6.5 mm cancellous screws is more effective than osteosynthesis using two or four 3.5 mm screws: with 6.5 mm screws, a load of 40–56 % more than 3.5 mm screws was required to cause system failure [23]. In Hoffa fractures the direction of the screws can change the mechanical stability. Screws placed from anterior to posterior are used to fix coronal fractures. This direction is usually preferred for an easy surgical

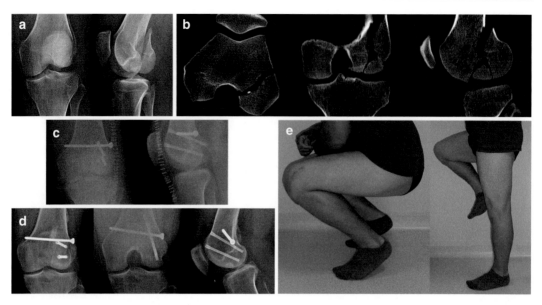

Fig. 4.3 Hoffa fracture. Case example of 35-year-old male. (**a**, **b**). X-rays and CT demonstrate type I Hoffa fracture of the lateral femoral condyle of the left femur. (**c**). Open reduction and fixation with two anteroposterior 4.3 mm compression screws and a 4.5 mm latero-medial cortical screw. (**d–e**). Four-year follow-up. Fracture healed without any sign of necrosis or arthritis. Full range of motion of the knee

approach, visualization, and screws placement. However, posterior-to-anterior screws provide better mechanical strength during loading [22]. In case of intra-articular screw placement, the screw heads must be recessed beneath the articular surface. The effects of the cartilage defects created with this technique are not known. To provide additional stability, a buttress plate can be used at the expense of additional soft tissue dissection along the posterior femur [41, 44].

Several authors report the arthroscopically assisted internal fixation for Hoffa fractures with good early results. Reduced soft tissue dissection, blood loss, operative time, and a faster recovery time compared with open procedure are the potential advantages of this technique. However, there is no evidence to suggest that arthroscopy may improve the treatment of these fractures [41, 44].

4.11 Blade Plate

Blade plate is a monoblock, preshaped implant that is adapted to the anatomy of the distal femur. In addition to extra-articular fractures (AO type A), blade plate is indicated in case of sagittal unicondylar fractures or supracondylar

and intercondylar fractures. The system is very stable, allowing compression of the epiphyseal-metaphyseal fracture site [2, 13]. Mechanically, the implant functions like a dynamic tension band creating a medial compression. In the osteoporotic bone, the placement of the blade can be traumatic and have little resistance to breakage [2, 13]. A supplemental medial fixation can be used in case of comminuted metaphyseal fractures with bone loss to prevent varus collapse [7]. Care is needed to ensure that screws do not interfere with subsequent implant placement. After securing the articular part, the extra-articular component of the fracture is addressed.

4.12 Dynamic Compression Plate

Besides extra-articular fractures, the classic indications are sagittal unicondylar fractures or supra- and intercondylar fractures. Epiphyseal fixation is obtained by a single lag screw which the plate pivots upon for sagittal adjustment. The implant has a 95° angle between the plate and the screw. This angle facilitates frontal placement and positions the epiphyseal screw parallel to the

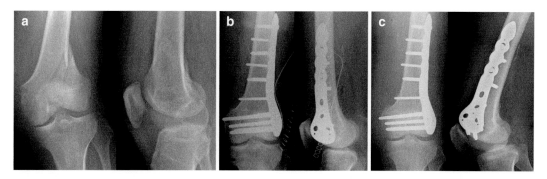

Fig. 4.4 Plate case.(**a**). AO 33-C1 fracture of the left femur in a 74-year-old man. (**b**). ORIF with a locking plate. (**c**). Six-month follow-up fracture healed

joint. This implant has the advantage of being fairly easy to position, because the lag screw is cannulated and having a good resistance to screw failure [2, 13]. However, the lag screw hole is large (~12.5 mm Ø) and can determine many problems for new fixation due a bone loss in case of implant revision.

4.13   Locking Compression Plate

Indications to use a locking compression plate are extra-articular fractures, sagittal unicondylar fractures, or supra- and intercondylar fractures. Locking compression plates have many advantages compared to dynamic compression plate: screw locking minimizes the compressive forces exerted by the plate to the bone and thus avoids disturbance of the bone blood supply [15, 33]; the system works as flexible elastic fixation that stimulates callus formation; precise anatomical shape allows using these plates as a "reduction mold," molding the bone to the plate and preventing primary dislocation of the fracture caused by inexact contouring of a normal plate; these plates also allow a better distribution of the angular and axial loading around the plate [15, 33].

The locking plate can be used with a classic open procedure when there is an intra-articular involvement, or with a minimally invasive approach. A combination of minimally invasive proximal diaphyseal fixation with an open distal internal fixation can be adopted to manage multi-fragmentary articular fractures. A potential disadvantage is the lack of epiphyseal compression with locking screws. To avoid this problem, com-

pression screws can be inserted through the plate first to achieve an optimal fracture reduction and then changed with locking screws. Another option is to use a King Tong clamp to compress the plate to the bone surface. Provisional K-wires inserted through the plate can help to position and maintain the implant in the correct place. The implant is finally fixed with locking screws (Fig. 4.4). Supplemental medial or anteromedial fixation can be considered in fractures with increased risk of failure with lateral-locked plating (i.e., open comminuted metaphyseal fractures with bone loss) in order to prevent varus collapse [7, 34].

4.14   Retrograde Nails

Retrograde intramedullary nailing allows fracture stabilization with minimal soft tissue and periosteal disruption around the fracture site. The classic indication is extra-articular fracture. However, the recent improvement in implant design and instrumentation makes the nail a reliable indication for selected intra-articular distal femoral fractures [7, 17]. The new nail generations allow the placement of interlocking screws, creating a fixed angle implant particularly useful in the osteoporotic bone and in short condylar fragments. Moreover, many interlocking screws within a few centimeters to the nail end can be implanted; in this way also, very far distal fractures can be treated with retrograde intramedullary nail (Fig. 4.5) [7].

In case of intra-articular fracture, nailing the distal femoral fractures can be technically

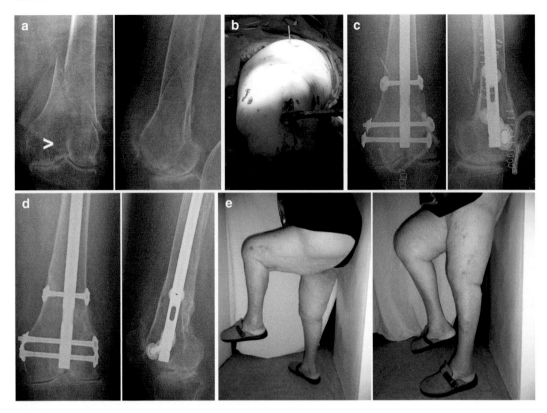

Fig. 4.5 Retrograde nail case. (**a**). AO 33-C1 fracture of the left femur in a 64-year-old woman with BMI 33 affected by severe osteoporosis and Crohn's disease. (>) shows the intercondylar fracture line. (**b**). Intraoperative. A retrograde nail was implanted through a minimally invasive approach. (**c**). X-rays postoperative. The articular fragments were fixed first with a bicondylar screw. The retrograde nailing was then implanted and the proximal bicondylar screw allowed to achieve a good compression of the metaphyseal fragments. (**d, e**). Six-month follow-up. Fracture healed without any malalignment. Good knee range of motion

demanding. An accurate preoperative planning is necessary to evaluate the fracture pattern: number and dislocation of the articular fragments and their length in relation to the nail and the possibility of using lag screws or condyle screws to fix the condylar fragment before nailing should be taken in account. In particular, the multiple anterior to posterior screws used to fix coronal plane fractures could block the distal interlocking screw, so they must be carefully planned before the nail passage. Moreover, nail insertion depth must be carefully determined: overseating a nail could limit interlocking options, while underseating a nail, leaving it prominent in the joint, can lead to patellofemoral pain and articular erosion [7].

Standard length of retrograde intramedullary nails extends to the lesser trochanter to minimize stress on the subtrochanteric region. A short supracondylar nail should be long enough to allow the placement of two interlocking screws in the proximal fragment [17]. However, a long nail is advised for several reasons: prevention of stress fractures at the tip of the short nail, increased working length of the nail and consequently micromotion that helps fracture healing, and increased nail stability because of the contact with the isthmus [7].

4.15　External Fixator

External fixation has a limited rule in the treatment of distal intra-articular femoral fractures. This fixation system is indicated in two different scenarios:

- Temporary bridging external fixation (TBEF) in damage orthopedic control (DOC)
- Definitive external fixation in severe open fractures and in metaphyseal comminution

Although surgical technique of the TBEF is not as challenging as the definitive one, the surgeon must follow precise rules to avoid acute and chronic complications.

Three factors need to be considered:

- Pin placement
- Pin linkage
- Correct deformity

Pin placement requires the knowledge of cross-sectional limb anatomy to avoid neurovascular injury [6] and intra-articular pin penetration [26]. Anterior diaphyseal femoral pins have been used since they are easier to implant compared to lateral and facilitate patient nursing. Furthermore, anterior femoral pin placement has been recommended because of preservation of the lateral cortex for definitive screw fixation through a plate or nail. Beltran et al. in an anatomic study defined the safe zone for anterior pin placement. Based on the distance between the last crossing femoral nerve branch and the superior reflection of the knee joint, the average safe zone corridor for anterior external fixator pin placement is approximately 20 cm, with the absolute narrowest zone identified as 12 cm. The upper limit is 5.8 cm below the lesser trochanter and the lower is 7.5 cm above the proximal pole of the patella [6]. Lateral pin placement reduces neurovascular lesions, the extensor mechanism, and knee joint penetration. Mercer et al., in a biomechanical study, compared the relative stiffness (varus, valgus, and axial loading) of four common external fixation configurations used to span and stabilize the knee after knee dislocation [28]. The four configurations evaluated were anterior femoral pins with monotube, anterolateral femoral pins with monotube, anterolateral femoral pins with two connecting rods, and hinged ring fixator. The authors concluded that the stiffest construct for external fixation is achieved with anterior lateral configuration on the femur and two connecting rods due to the biplanar nature of the construct. Strebe at al. compared the mechanical benefits of three strategies that are commonly used to increase knee-spanning external fixator stiffness (resistance to deformation): double stacking, cross-linking, and the use of an oblique pin. The authors concluded that only double stacking increased stiffness in all four testing modalities ($p < 0.05$) [40].

In hemodynamically unstable patients, the primary goal to achieve with TBEF is restoring the limb length. In the hemodynamically stable patients, a complete realignment should be obtained. A shortening of 1 cm can be acceptable until 2 or 3 weeks because, if the definitive surgery is delayed for a longer period, it is very difficult to restore the normal limb length [31]. An overdistraction should be applied at fracture site to avoid this problem. However, if the local limb blood supply is critical due to a vascular lesion, an overdistraction could be dangerous for the epiphyseal fragments vascularity [31].

The use of external fixation as definitive treatment is very rare. Distal pins and fiches placement can result in septic arthritis due to iatrogenic penetration of the knee capsule. However, the incidence is unknown in the distal femur [26]. Minimally invasive approach to reduce the articular fracture and fixation with screws should be performed before external fixation. Even if divergent olive wires through the condyles provide good compression and stability, indirect reduction of the epiphyseal fragments by ligamentotaxis can be difficult to achieve especially in type C2 and type C3 fractures [4].

4.16 Postoperative Regimen

Postoperative management depends on different factors: fracture pattern, implant used, stability of the fracture fixation construct, concomitant injuries, bone quality, and patient compliance. The wounds should be checked regularly and the sutures removed after 2 weeks from surgery. An adequate pharmaceutical and mechanical thrombosis prophylaxis must be administered.

Rehabilitation should be followed by a physical therapist under surgeon supervision. In some cases it is appropriate to protect the fracture from varus and valgus stresses using a hinged knee brace. Knee motion should begin immediately whenever possible to prevent stiffness and loss of function. A continuous passive motion machine can be used to facilitate a gradual advancement in knee range of motion. Quadriceps and hamstring strengthening should be encouraged early after the operation, helping in maximizing the functional recovery. Gait training can be initiated on day 1 in compliant patients. In intra-articular fracture, nonweight-bearing or weight-bearing restriction should be held until 10–12 weeks postoperatively, or until fracture healing is visible radiographically. Clinical and radiographic examinations are typically taken at 4–6 weeks intervals until fracture healing and the patients are able to walk without discomfort [7, 17].

4.17 Complications

The main complications of distal femoral fracture are delayed union or nonunion, deep infection, malalignment, and arthrofibrosis. Osteoarthritis is the most frequent long-term complication, but the incidence has not been reported in the literature [36]. The overall rate of healing problems, including delayed union, nonunion, implant revision, or secondary bone grafting, ranges from 0 to 32 % [18]. Ricci et al. in a retrospective study analyzed the risk factors for reoperation to promote union, deep infection, and implant failure of 335 distal femoral fractures (AO 33-A or 33-C, 33 % open) treated with lateral-locked plates [35]. Reoperation rate was 19 %. The following factors were significantly associated to reoperation risk: open fracture, diabetes, smoking, high BMI, short proximal plate length, and young age. The authors postulated that young age is a risk factor due to the higher-energy mechanisms of trauma. Deep infection occurred in 5 % of fractures from the entire series. The authors identified open fracture, obesity, diabetes, and stainless steel plate as being associated with deep infection. Implant failure occurred in 7 % of the cases and most failures

occurred within the zone of the proximal fragment. When shorter plates (nine holes) were used, there was a 14 % failure rate compared with 1 % failure with longer plates. Smith et al. reported loss of reduction as the most frequent complication, more commonly in varus/valgus than in flexion/extension and even less common in external rotation [38]. In case of metaphyseal comminution, a varus collapse was observed [20].

In the literature many studies report the management of nonunion of the distal femur. However, the guidelines are not standardized. Ebraheim et al. in a systematic review noted that the most common definitive treatment was fixed angle plating combined with cancellous autografting [12]. The authors concluded that this treatment had a successful union rate of 97.4 % and the average time to heal was 7.8 months. In the osteoporotic bone or mechanically atrophic unstable nonunion, opposite allograft cortical struts or locking plate are useful to stabilize the implant (Figs. 4.6 and 4.7).

In case of malalignment after bone healing, osteotomy, immediate correction, and fixation with a plate should be planned. Limb shortening more than 1.5 cm associated with an angulation more than 7–10° on coronal plane can be managed with external fixation [7, 17].

Deep infection is managed with appropriate antibiotic administration after harvesting samples for microbiological culture, implant removal, debridement of all the infected bone and soft tissue, and one- or two-staged fixation procedure [27].

Posttraumatic osteoarthritis can be managed with osteotomy, unicompartmental knee arthroplasty (UKA), and total knee arthroplasty (TKA), according to the joint morphology and involvement of one or more knee compartments. Malunion, intra-articular osseous defects, limb malalignment, retained internal fixation devices, and damaged surrounding soft tissues may decrease the functional outcome of prosthesis in these patients [32].

4.18 Results

In the literature many studies have been reported for the treatment of intra-articular/distal femoral fracture with a single implant (screws, plate,

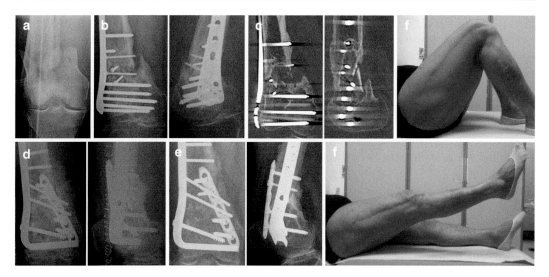

Fig. 4.6 Nonunion case. (**a**). AO 33-C3 fracture of the left femur in a 71-year-old woman. (**b, c**). X-rays and CT scan at 1-year follow-up after ORIF with a locking plate. Atrophic nonunion with bone loss at the medial side. (**d**). X-rays postoperative. Internal fixation with blade plate, anteromedial 4.5 mm locking plate and composite graft (see Fig. 4.7). (**e, f**). Six-month follow-up. Fracture healed with good knee range of motion

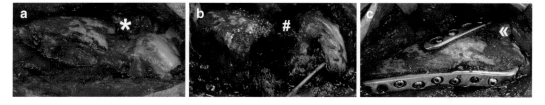

Fig. 4.7 Intraoperative of the nonunion case. (**a**). Plate removed. (*) Nonunion of the metaphyseal part. (**b**). Debridement of the lesion and residual bone loss (#). (**c**). Internal fixation with blade plate, anteromedial 4.5 mm locking plate and RIA graft (reamer irrigator aspirator), bone substitute, and BMP-7. RIA graft (reamer irrigator aspirator), bone substitute and BMP-7 (<<)

nail, etc.). However, there is a lack of comparative studies and in particular of prospective studies. Bel et al. reported the results of the surgical treatment of 163 unicondylar fractures (82 % AO B2, 18 % AO B3) at a mean follow-up of 7 years. In this multicenter study, 23 % of B1 fractures were treated with a lateral buttress plate and a medial buttress plate was used in 4 % of B2 fractures [5]. All the B3 fractures were fixed only with screws; anterior lag screws were used in 78 % of cases, and direct posterior-to-anterior screw fixation was performed in 15 % of cases. The authors observed intra-articular malunion in 27 % of cases due to an insufficient reduction, valgus-varus deformity in 10 %, flexion-recurvatum deformity in 5 %, and 12 % of osteoarthritis. The authors concluded that a correct approach can influence the ability to achieve anatomic reduction and stable fixation. For the treatment of B3 fracture, a posterior/posteromedial approach should be advised to perform direct posterior-to-anterior screw fixation. A biomechanical study demonstrated that direct posterior-to-anterior screw fixation via posterior approach is stronger than anterior lag screw fixation [22].

Garnavos et al., in a prospective study, evaluated 17 patients affected by AO 33 type C fracture treated with retrograde nail and bicondylar screws [16]. No case of malunion, nonunion, and infection were reported, and good functional and clinical scores were recorded. The authors concluded that the association between retrograde nail and a compression condylar bolt allowed good functional results. In a retrospective series of 115 fractures, Hierholzer et al. compared retrograde nail (*n*=59) and minimally invasive locking plate (*n*=56) [19]. They did not note any difference in terms of functional and radiological outcomes between intra-articular and extra-articular fractures. Differences between groups for type A fractures were statistically not significant. Statistical analysis for type C fractures between the two groups was not possible since in type C2 and C3 fractures, only LISS plating was performed. Thomson et al., in a small series of 22 patients with a mean 80 month follow-up, compared the clinical, functional, and radiographic outcomes of ORIF versus limited open reduction and retrograde nailing in the treatment of distal femoral fractures (AO type C) [42]. In the plate group, they observed 42 % malalignment, 33 % nonunion, and 25 % infection with 67 % of cases that required a subsequent bone-grafting procedure. Instead in the retrograde nail group, they recorded no cases of malunion and infection, while a nonunion rate of 9 % was reported. Ehlinger et al. proposed the indications for each technique: the plate can manage all fractures, while retrograde nailing is better to treat extra-articular fractures [13].

Arazi et al. reported the results of Ilizarov external fixation for the acute treatment of severely comminuted extra-articular and intercondylar fractures of the distal femur [4]. A total of 14 consecutive patients with complex fractures were treated and evaluated at a mean follow-up of 14 months. There were three type A3, two type C2, and nine type C3 fractures according to the AO classification. Fractures healed in 13/14 cases with excellent or good results in 64 % of the patients. Limited knee flexion was seen in most patients. The mean range of flexion at final follow-up was 105° (35°–130°). The limitation of movement was greatest in patients with a type C3 fracture. El Tantawy et al. applied the concept of distraction osteogenesis for the treatment of 17 comminuted distal femoral fractures (10 type C2 and 7 type C3.2 fractures) [14]. The procedure included initial percutaneous fixation of the articular fragments by inter-fragmentary screws, acute shortening using an Ilizarov fixator, followed by gradual re-distraction to compensate the shortening. All fractures healed in an average of 4.5 months, and the functional results were excellent in 3 cases, good in 12, and fair in 2 patients. Complications included pin track infection in eight cases (47 %) and superficial wound infection in three cases (18 %). Hutson and Zych reported the results of the treatment of 16 fractures (1 type C3.1, 1 type C3.2, 14 type C3.3); 12 out of 16 were open fracture [21]. Limited open fixation of the joint surface and tensioned wire circular external fixation of the metaphysis and shaft was the surgical strategy. The average follow-up was 35 months (range, 14–60 months). All the fracture healed. There were two excellent, nine good, and five fair results. Two patients had delayed bone grafting for delayed union. Five patients required a quadricepsplasty. One patient developed septic arthritis and another developed osteomyelitis. The authors concluded that limited internal fixation and tensioned wire external fixation have equivalent results to other methods but have a higher incidence of infection and complications. Joint motion is retarded by binding of the soft tissues with fixation wires and pins. The technique is recommended only for salvage of severely comminuted and open fractures of the distal femur with extensive soft tissue injury [21].

References

1. Agarwal S, Giannoudis PV, Smith RM (2004) Cruciate fracture of the distal femur: the double Hoffa fracture. Injury 35:828–830
2. Albert MJ (1997) Supracondylar fractures of the femur. J Am Acad Orthop Surg 5:163–171
3. Arastu MH, Kokke MC, Duffy PJ et al (2013) Coronal plane partial articular fractures of the distal femoral condyle: current concepts in management. Bone Joint J 95-B:1165–1171
4. Arazi M, Memik R, Ogun TC et al (2001) Ilizarov external fixation for severely comminuted supracondylar and intercondylar fractures of the distal femur. J Bone Joint Surg Br 83:663–667
5. Bel JC, Court C, Cogan A et al (2014) Unicondylar fractures of the distal femur. Orthop Traumatol Surg Res 100:873–877
6. Beltran MJ, Collinge CA, Patzkowski JC et al (2012) The safe zone for external fixator pins in the femur. J Orthop Trauma 26:643–647

7. Beltran MJ, Gary JL, Collinge CA (2015) Management of distal femur fractures with modern plates and nails: state of the art. J Orthop Trauma 29:165–172
8. Butt MS, Krikler SJ, Ali MS (1996) Displaced fractures of the distal femur in elderly patients. Operative versus non-operative treatment. J Bone Joint Surg Br 78:110–114
9. Chiron P, Giordano G, Besombes C et al (2005) Ostéosynthèse par la vis-plaque condylienne de Judet-Chiron. À propos d'une série continue de 364 fractures récentes. Springer, Paris
10. Court-Brown CM, Caesar B (2006) Epidemiology of adult fractures: a review. Injury 37:691–697
11. Dhillon MS, Mootha AK, Bali K et al (2012) Coronal fractures of the medial femoral condyle: a series of 6 cases and review of literature. Musculoskelet Surg 96:49–54
12. Ebraheim NA, Martin A, Sochacki KR, Liu J (2013) Nonunion of distal femoral fractures: a systematic review. Orthop Surg 5:46–50
13. Ehlinger M, Ducrot G, Adam P et al (2012) Distal femur fractures. Surgical techniques and a review of the literature. Orthop Traumatol Surg Res 99:353–360
14. El-Tantawy A, Atef A (2015) Comminuted distal femur closed fractures: a new application of the Ilizarov concept of compression-distraction. Eur J Orthop Surg Traumatol 25:555–562
15. Frigg R (2003) Development of the locking compression plate. Injury 34(Suppl 2):B6–B10
16. Garnavos C, Lygdas P, Lasanianos NG (2012) Retrograde nailing and compression bolts in the treatment of type C distal femoral fractures. Injury 43:1170–1175
17. Gwathmey FW Jr, Jones-Quaidoo SM, Kahler D et al (2010) Distal femoral fractures: current concepts. J Am Acad Orthop Surg 18:597–607
18. Henderson CE, Kuhl LL, Fitzpatrick DC et al (2013) Locking plates for distal femur fractures: is there a problem with fracture healing? J Orthop Trauma 25(Suppl 1):S8–S14
19. Hierholzer C, von Ruden C, Potzel T et al (2011) Outcome analysis of retrograde nailing and less invasive stabilization system in distal femoral fractures: a retrospective analysis. Indian J Orthop 45:243–250
20. Hoffmann MF, Jones CB, Sietsema DL et al (2013) Clinical outcomes of locked plating of distal femoral fractures in a retrospective cohort. J Orthop Surg Res 8:43
21. Hutson JJ Jr, Zych GA (2000) Treatment of comminuted intraarticular distal femur fractures with limited internal and external tensioned wire fixation. J Orthop Trauma 14:405–413
22. Jarit GJ, Kummer FJ, Gibber MJ et al (2006) A mechanical evaluation of two fixation methods using cancellous screws for coronal fractures of the lateral condyle of the distal femur (OTA type 33B). J Orthop Trauma 20:273–276
23. Khalafi A, Hazelwood S, Curtiss S et al (2008) Fixation of the femoral condyles: a mechanical comparison of small and large fragment screw fixation. J Trauma 64:740–744
24. Letenneur J, Labour PE, Rogez JM et al (1978) Hoffa's fractures. Report of 20 cases (author's transl). Ann Chir 32:213–219
25. Link BC, Babst R (2012) Current concepts in fractures of the distal femur. Acta Chir Orthop Traumatol Cech 79:11–20
26. Lowery K, Dearden P, Sherman K et al (2015) Cadaveric analysis of capsular attachments of the distal femur related to pin and wire placement. Injury 46:970–974
27. McNally MA, Small JO, Tofighi HG et al (1993) Two-stage management of chronic osteomyelitis of the long bones. The Belfast technique. J Bone Joint Surg Br 75:375–380
28. Mercer D, Firoozbakhsh K, Prevost M et al (2010) Stiffness of knee-spanning external fixation systems for traumatic knee dislocations: a biomechanical study. J Orthop Trauma 24:693–696
29. Muller E, Nazarian S, Koch P et al (1990) The comprehensive classification of fracture of long bone. Springer, Berlin
30. Nork SE, Segina DN, Aflatoon K et al (2005) The association between supracondylar-intercondylar distal femoral fractures and coronal plane fractures. J Bone Joint Surg Am 87:564–569
31. Oh JK, Hwang JH, Sahu D et al (2011) Complication rate and pitfalls of temporary bridging external fixator in periarticular communited fractures. Clin Orthop Surg 3:62–68
32. Papadopoulos EC, Parvizi J, Lai CH et al (2002) Total knee arthroplasty following prior distal femoral fracture. Knee 9:267–274
33. Perren SM (2002) Evolution of the internal fixation of long bone fractures. The scientific basis of biological internal fixation: choosing a new balance between stability and biology. J Bone Joint Surg Br 84:1093–1110
34. Prayson MJ, Datta DK, Marshall MP (2001) Mechanical comparison of endosteal substitution and lateral plate fixation in supracondylar fractures of the femur. J Orthop Trauma 15:96–100
35. Ricci WM, Streubel PN, Morshed S et al (2014) Risk factors for failure of locked plate fixation of distal femur fractures: an analysis of 335 cases. J Orthop Trauma 28:83–89
36. Rodriguez EK, Boulton C, Weaver MJ et al (2014) Predictive factors of distal femoral fracture nonunion after lateral locked plating: a retrospective multicenter case-control study of 283 fractures. Injury 45:554–559
37. Seinsheimer F 3rd (1980) Fractures of the distal femur. Clin Orthop Relat Res 153:169–179
38. Smith TO, Hedges C, MacNair R et al (2009) The clinical and radiological outcomes of the LISS plate for distal femoral fractures: a systematic review. Injury 40:1049–1063
39. Starr AJ, Jones AL, Reinert CM (1999) The "swashbuckler": a modified anterior approach for fractures of the distal femur. J Orthop Trauma 13:138–140
40. Strebe S, Kim H, Russell JP et al (2014) Analysis of strategies to increase external fixator stiffness: is double stacking worth the cost? Injury 45:1049–1053

41. Tetsunaga T, Sato T, Shiota N et al (2013) Posterior buttress plate with locking compression plate for Hoffa fracture. J Orthop Sci 18:798–802

42. Thomson AB, Driver R, Kregor PJ et al (2008) Long-term functional outcomes after intra-articular distal femur fractures: ORIF versus retrograde intramedullary nailing. Orthopedics 31:748–750

43. Trillat A, Dejour H, Bost J et al (1975) Unicondylar fractures of the femur. Rev Chir Orthop Reparatrice Appar Mot 61:611–626

44. White EA, Matcuk GR, Schein A et al (2015) Coronal plane fracture of the femoral condyles: anatomy, injury patterns, and approach to management of the Hoffa fragment. Skeletal Radiol 44:37–43

Management of Simple Proximal Tibia Fractures (Schatzker Types I–IV)

5

Davide Edoardo Bonasia

Abstract

Tibial plateau fractures constitute approximately 1 % of all fractures. Approximately 5–10 % of tibial plateau fractures are sports related, and proximal tibial fractures are especially common in high-energy sport injuries (i.e., skiing, football, rugby, etc.). The lateral tibial plateau is affected in 55–70 % of the cases, the medial plateau in 10–23 %, and both plateaux in 10–30 %. In this chapter, the treatment of simple tibial plateau fractures (type I to IV according to Schatzker's classification) will be discussed, including conservative treatment, arthroscopic reduction and internal fixation (ARIF), and open reduction and internal fixation (ORIF).

5.1 Epidemiology

Tibial plateau fractures constitute approximately 1 % of all fractures [1]. Approximately 5–10 % of tibial plateau fractures are sports related, and proximal tibial fractures are especially common in high-energy sporting injuries (i.e., skiing, football, rugby, etc.) [1, 2]. The lateral tibial plateau is affected in 55–70 % of the cases, the medial plateau in 10–23 %, and both plateaux in 10–30 % [3].

Meniscal tears can be associated with tibial plateau fractures in 42.2 % of the cases, while anterior cruciate ligament (ACL) tears in 21.3 %

[4]. Neurovascular structures can be damaged as well, mostly the popliteal artery in complex fractures and the common peroneal nerve in lateral plateau fractures due to direct impaction (valgus force).

5.2 Traumatic Mechanism

Although tibial plateau fractures were originally called "bumper" or "fender" fractures, only 25 % of these fractures result from impact with automobile bumpers. The most common mechanism of injury involves axial loading (i.e., fall from a height). Other patterns of injury result from laterally directed forces or from a twisting injury. In all cases, force is transmitted through the femoral condyles onto the medial or lateral tibial plateaux. While split fractures are common in

D.E. Bonasia, MD
Department of Orthopaedics and Traumatology, University of Torino, Mauriziano "Umberto I" Hospital, Via Lamarmora 26, Torino 10128, Italy
e-mail: davidebonasia@virgilio.it

© Springer International Publishing Switzerland 2016
F. Castoldi, D.E. Bonasia (eds.), *Fractures Around the Knee*, Fracture Management Joint by Joint, DOI 10.1007/978-3-319-28806-2_5

the younger population, depression fractures are commonly seen in older, osteoporotic patients.

5.3 Clinical Examination

Clinically, the traumatic mechanism should be investigated and a dislocation ruled out. The knee is usually swollen and painful and the physical examination should be mainly focused on the neurovascular evaluation and possible associated lesions. Palpation of the bony structures around the knee can help identify the location of the fracture/s. Stability maneuvers must be carried out under anesthesia, before surgery. In case of unclear diagnosis after the x-rays, aspiration of blood with fat droplets from the joint may be helpful to confirm the diagnosis of intra-articular fracture and justify further investigation.

5.4 Imaging and Preoperative Work-Up

For a correct assessment of the fracture type and degree of displacement, the preoperative work-up must include anteroposterior (AP) and lateral x-ray views (sometimes oblique views) as well as a CT scan of the knee. Magnetic resonance

imaging (MRI) is not routinely required but may be useful when associated ligamentous injuries are suspected, even though ligament reconstruction is usually delayed after fracture healing.

5.5 Classification

A correct classification of the fracture is mandatory for the decision making and to assess the prognosis. Many classification systems are available for tibial plateau fractures (i.e., Hohl, Moore, Honkonen and Jarvinen, AO, etc.), but Schatzker's classification has the advantages of handiness as well as a good correlation with severity, treatment, and prognosis of the fracture [3]. Type I is a wedge fracture of the lateral hemiplateau, without articular depression (Fig. 5.1). Type II is a wedge fracture of the lateral hemiplateau associated with articular depression (Fig. 5.2). Type III is an isolated articular depression fracture involving the lateral plateau (Figs. 5.3 and 5.4). Type IV is a medial tibial plateau fracture, most likely associated with tibial eminence fracture (Fig. 5.5). Type V is a bicondylar tibial fracture, without metaphyseal involvement. Type VI is a unicondylar or bicondylar tibial fracture, with metaphyseal involvement.

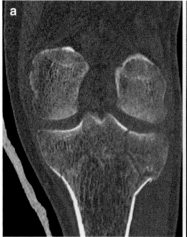 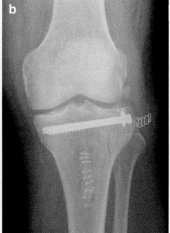 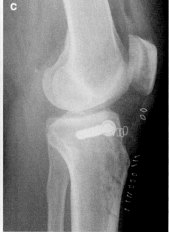

Fig. 5.1 Schatzker type I fracture (split fracture lateral). (**a**) Coronal CT scan; (**b**) postoperative AP view; (**c**) postoperative lateral view. The procedure consisted of arthroscopically assisted reduction and percutaneous fixation with cannulated screws

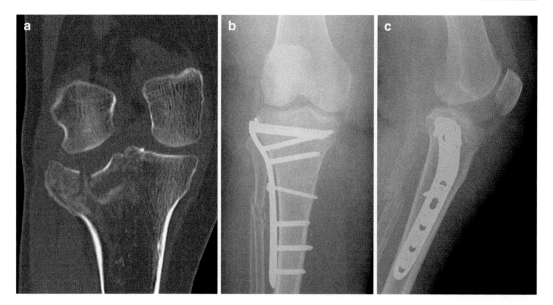

Fig. 5.2 Schatzker type II fracture (split/depression fracture lateral). (**a**) Coronal CT scan; (**b**) postoperative AP view; (**c**) postoperative lateral view. The procedure consisted of open reduction and internal fixation with plate

5.6   Indications

The management of the fracture depends on several factors and these include (1) fracture configuration, (2) concomitant soft tissue injury, (3) patient's age and activity level, and (4) bone quality.

Nondisplaced and minimally displaced/depressed fractures or displaced fractures in arthritic knees can be treated conservatively or with percutaneous fixation. Displaced or depressed fractures with a step-off greater than 5 mm require reduction and internal fixation. There are inadequate data on the amount of articular depression and displacement that may lead to post-traumatic arthritis [2]. Some authors suggested that fracture displacement ranging from 4 to 10 mm should be treated conservatively, whereas others state that surgery is essential for articular depression greater than 3 or 4 mm. In case of nondisplaced but unstable fractures, rigid internal fixation may still be considered for active patients and athletes in whom early range of motion is a priority [2]. Five millimeter can be considered a reasonable cutoff for surgical indication.

When a conservative treatment is indicated, the management depends on the location and stability of the fracture. For unstable fractures involving the weight-bearing surface of the plateau, the knee is immobilized in a hinged knee brace for 2 weeks, and then 30° of ROM are allowed every week. Weight bearing is allowed at 3 months. In case of stable fractures, ROM 0–90° can be allowed immediately. In case of fractures not involving the weight-bearing area of the plateau, early weight bearing can be allowed.

Arthroscopic reduction and internal fixation (ARIF) is indicated in Schatzker types I, II, and III (Figs. 5.1, 5.3, and 5.4), when the displacement is more than 5 mm, in compliant patients and in non-arthritic knees. However, in some Schatzker type II fractures, if the bone quality is poor or the wedge fragment is comminuted, open reduction and internal fixation (ORIF) with plating is recommended (Fig. 5.2).

Arthroscopic-assisted techniques have been described also for Schatzker type IV fractures (Fig. 5.5). These fractures usually result from high-energy traumas, with soft tissue injuries (skin, ligaments, and capsule), and are more difficult to reduce by external maneuvers. For these reasons, in these cases, ORIF is recommended, also to avoid possible arthroscopic fluid leakage in the soft tissues.

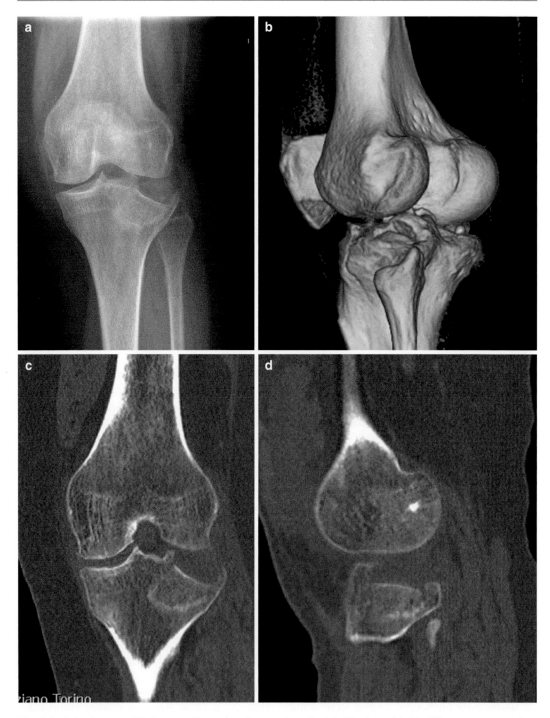

Fig. 5.3 Schatzker type III fracture (depression fracture lateral). (**a**) AP view; (**b**) 3D CT scan reconstruction; (**c**) coronal CT scan; (**d**) sagittal CT scan

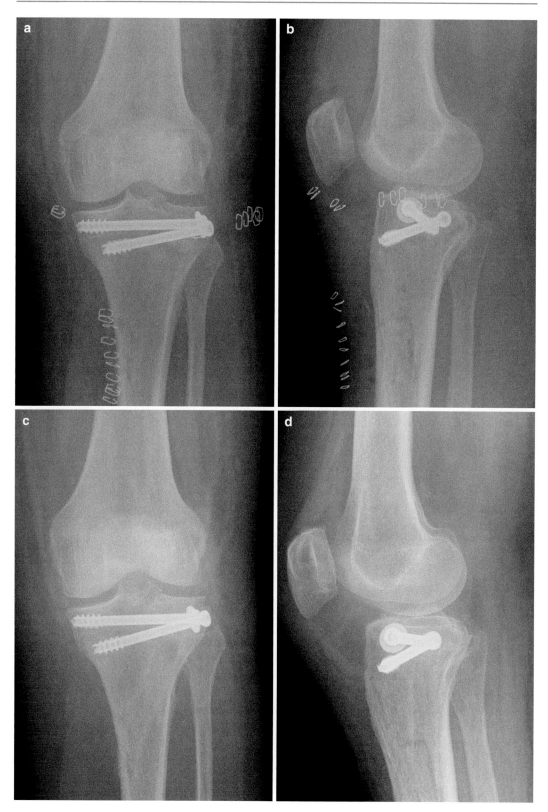

Fig. 5.4 Postoperative imaging of the case shown in Fig. 5.3. (**a**) Early postoperative AP view; (**b**) early postoperative lateral view; (**c**) 6-month postoperative AP view; (**d**) 6-month postoperative lateral view. The procedure consisted of arthroscopically assisted reduction and percutaneous fixation with cannulated screws

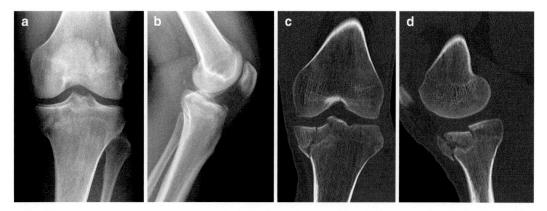

Fig. 5.5 Schatzker type IV fracture (medial plateau fracture). (**a**) AP view; (**b**) lateral view; (**c**) coronal CT scan; (**d**) sagittal CT scan

Fracture type (Schatzker classification)	Treatment
Type I (split fracture lateral)	ARIF and percutaneous lag screw fixation
Type II (split/depression fracture lateral)	ARIF and percutaneous lag screw fixation versus ORIF and plating (if poor bone quality or high comminution of the wedge fragment)
Type III (depression fracture lateral)	ARIF and percutaneous lag screw fixation
Type IV (medial fracture with tibial eminence avulsion)	ORIF and plating versus ARIF and percutaneous lag screw fixation (if low-energy trauma and isolated involvement of the medial plateau, either wedge or depressed fragment)

5.7 Surgical Techniques

5.7.1 Arthroscopic Reduction and Internal Fixation (ARIF)

The patient is positioned supine in general or spinal anesthesia, with the tourniquet placed on the proximal thigh. Preoperative antibiotic prophylaxis is administered IV. Knee stability is evaluated under anesthesia.

The main surgeon is on the side of the affected limb, while the C-arm and the arthroscopic screen are on the contralateral side. A specifically designed instrumentation is required (Fig. 5.6). Arthroscopic examination is performed using gravity inflow, through classical anteromedial and anterolateral portals. The hemarthrosis is drained and any osteochondral fragments removed. The degree of fracture depression and soft tissues injury is assessed.

A longitudinal 3 cm skin incision is made on the medial aspect of the tibia, starting 10 cm from the articular surface and extended distally (Fig. 5.7). A cortical window (10 × 20 mm) is opened on the medial tibia and a hollow trephine cutter (10 mm diameter), with a saw-toothed tip, is introduced in the tibia (Fig. 5.8).

Under fluoroscopic control (anteroposterior and lateral views), the edge of the cutter is placed 2 cm below the lateral plateau fracture (Fig. 5.8). A bone punch (9 mm diameter) is then inserted into the cutter and, with a hammer, the cancellous bone block (base 9 mm diameter, height about 100 mm) is impacted under the fracture to obtain an indirect reduction. If the articular surface is severely depressed, this procedure can be repeated placing the cutter in another direction, through the same window. The anatomical reconstruction of the articular surface is assessed arthroscopically (Fig. 5.9). Once the optimal reduction is achieved, the fracture is then fixed with two or three cancellous cannulated screws (6.5 mm) with washer, inserted percutaneously from lateral to medial and 1 cm under the articular surface. The cutter and the punch are then removed and the tibial cortex placed in situ. Neither iliac crest graft nor bone substitutes are used with this technique.

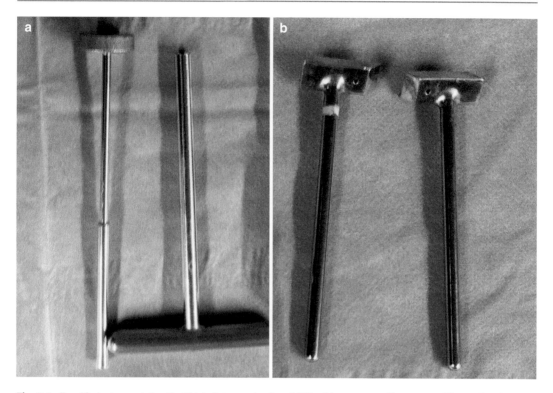

Fig. 5.6 Specific instrumentation for tibial plateau reduction. (**a**) Trephine cutter and bone tamp; (**b**) template for cortical window creation

In Schatzker type I fractures (wedge fractures, without articular surface depression), the elevation of the depressed surface is not required and, under arthroscopic control, the wedge fragment is usually reduced by external maneuvers. These include a digital compression on the wedge fragment that is usually distally displaced, a varus stress on the knee (playing on the ligamentotaxis by the articular capsule), and the use of a K wire, with a "joystick technique." Once the fracture is reduced and the articular surface restored, a percutaneous fixation with screws is performed, as previously described [5, 6].

5.7.2 Open Reduction and Internal Fixation (ORIF)

The patient position and preparation are as described for ARIF. Alternatively, the foot of the operating table can be dropped down (flexing the knee to 90°).

Both lateral hockey stick incision and lateral parapatellar longitudinal approaches can be used. The hockey stick incision has the advantage of an easier approach to the fracture, while the longitudinal incision does not interfere with subsequent total knee replacement.

The lateral hockey stick incision is started from the lateral epicondyle and extended distally to 2 cm below the Gerdy's tubercle. This incision can be extended proximally or distally according to the fracture's pattern. The iliotibial band is incised over the fracture site. The anterior compartment muscles are elevated off the proximal tibia with a Cobb elevator. An inframeniscal approach is used to reach the joint. The meniscocapsular detachment needs to be large enough to allow lateral meniscus elevation and lateral fragment opening. By opening the lateral fragment, the depressed portion of the articular surface is elevated, with a bone tamp, and auto- or allograft augmentation is performed. The lateral split fragment is reduced with the use of a reduction clamp,

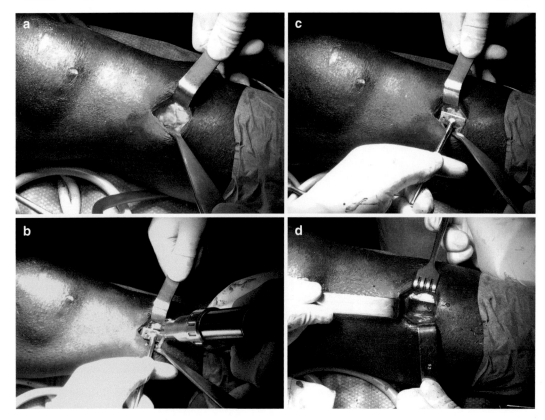

Fig. 5.7 Arthroscopically assisted reduction and fixation of tibial plateau fractures. (**a**) Anteromedial incision (approximately 10 cm distal to the articular surface); (**b**) template for cortical window creation; (**c**) cortical window creation with the oscillating saw; (**d**) window after removal of the cortex

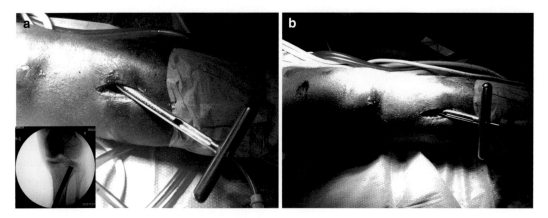

Fig. 5.8 Arthroscopically assisted reduction and fixation of tibial plateau fractures. (**a**) Trephine cutter placed 1 cm under the depressed fragment with the image intensifier; (**b**) bone tamp to reduce the depressed fragment

Fig. 5.9
Arthroscopically assisted reduction and fixation of tibial plateau fractures. (**a**) Arthroscopic image before fracture reduction; (**b**) arthroscopic image after fracture reduction

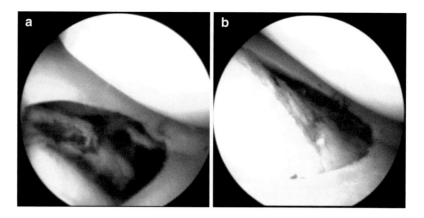

under direct visualization and image intensifier control. Temporary fixation is achieved with K wires. An L (or T)-shaped contoured 4.5 mm locking plate is used for final fixation (Fig. 5.2).

5.8 Postoperative Regimen

Immediate active motion 0–90° is allowed in a hinged knee brace. The brace is removed after 8 weeks and partial (or toe touch) weight bearing allowed after 8 weeks. Full weight is permitted 3 months after surgery.

5.9 Complications

The most common complications include [4]:

- Post-traumatic arthritis (26 %)
- Reduced range of motion (10 %)
- Loss of correction of more than 4 mm (1.5 %) and post-traumatic malalignment
- Deep infection (0.5 %)
- Deep venous thrombosis (0.3 %)
- Compartment syndrome (0.2 %)
- Peroneal nerve neuropraxia

5.10 Results

In a recent systematic review (19 articles, 609 patients), Chen et al. described that 90.5 % of the patients had classifications of good or excellent

clinical scores (Rasmussen score) and 90.9 % of the patients were satisfied with ARIF [4]. The authors concluded that ARIF is a reliable, effective, and safe method for the treatment of tibial plateau fractures.

No prospective randomized controlled studies comparing the clinical results of ARIF and ORIF are available. Only three retrospective studies (level III) comparing ARIF and ORIF [7–9] were published.

Dall'Oca et al. [8] compared 50 patients with tibial plateau fractures treated with ARIF with 50 patients treated with ORIF. The authors suggested that there were no differences between the two techniques for the treatment of Schatzker type I fractures. In the case of Schatzker type II, III, and IV fractures, the clinical outcomes were slightly in favor of ARIF (not statistically significant).

Ohdera et al. retrospectively evaluated 28 patients treated for tibial plateau fractures (19 ARIF and 9 ORIF). There was no significant difference between the groups in terms of duration of operation, postoperative flexion, and clinical results. In the ARIF group, however, the postoperative rehabilitation was easier and faster. Furthermore, 16 of 19 patients (84 %) in the ARIF group obtained an anatomical reduction (defined as <2 mm of residual displacement after surgery), whereas in the ORIF group, only 5 out of 9 patients (55 %) had an anatomical reduction [7].

Fowble et al. evaluated 23 patients with tibial plateau fractures (compression or split compression). Twelve patients were treated with ARIF and 11 with ORIF. In the ARIF group, all reductions were anatomic, whereas only 6 (55 %) of the ORIF patients had anatomical reductions initially. Faster recovery and earlier weight bearing were also noted for the ARIF group, compared with ORIF [9].

Studies with larger sample sizes and higher level of evidence are required to definitely assess a gold standard in the treatment of type I to IV Schatzker fractures.

References

1. Gill TJ, Moezzi DM, Oates KM, Sterett WI (2001) Arthroscopic reduction and internal fixation of tibial plateau fractures in skiing. Clin Orthop Relat Res 383:243–249
2. Lubowitz JH, Elson WS, Guttmann D (2004) Part I: arthroscopic management of tibial plateau fractures. Arthroscopy 20(10):1063–1070
3. Bonasia DE, Rossi R, Bardelli A (2005) Tibial plateau fractures. A review of classifications. Minerva Ortopedica e Traumatologica 56(5):457–463
4. Chen XZ, Liu CG, Chen Y, Wang LQ, Zhu QZ, Lin P (2015) Arthroscopy-assisted surgery for tibial plateau fractures. Arthroscopy 31(1):143–153
5. Rossi R, Bonasia DE, Blonna D, Assom M, Castoldi F (2008) Prospective follow-up of a simple arthroscopic-assisted technique for lateral tibial plateau fractures: results at 5 years. Knee 15(5): 378–383
6. Rossi R, Castoldi F, Blonna D, Marmotti A, Assom M (2006) Arthroscopic treatment of lateral tibial plateau fractures: a simple technique. Arthroscopy 22(6):678. e1–678.e6
7. Ohdera T, Tokunaga M, Hiroshima S, Yoshimoto E, Tokunaga J, Kobayashi A (2003) Arthroscopic management of tibial plateau fractures comparison with open reduction method. Arch Orthop Trauma Surg 123:489–493
8. Dall'Oca C, Maluta T, Lavini F, Bondi M, Micheloni GM, Bartolozzi P (2012) Tibial plateau fractures: compared outcomes between ARIF and ORIF. Strategies Trauma Limb Reconstr 7:163–175
9. Fowble CD, Zimmer JW, Schepsis AA (1993) The role of arthroscopy in the assessment and treatment of tibial plateau fractures. Arthroscopy 9:584–590

Management of Complex Proximal Tibia Fractures (Schatzker Types V and VI)

6

Jodi Siegel and Paul Tornetta III

Abstract

Complex tibial plateau fractures are challenging to manage successfully due to both the fracture and the associated soft tissue injury. Restoring length and alignment while avoiding complications is the goal of treatment. Meticulous soft tissue management and thoughtful surgical decision-making can result in good functional outcomes. Understanding the pathoanatomy of the fracture is important for selecting the method of fixation that will maintain the reduction until union.

6.1 Introduction

Tibial plateau fractures are injuries to the proximal tibia that include fractures of the articular surface. They represent a large spectrum of injuries in both complexity and severity. Successful management requires restoring the bony anatomy while respecting the surrounding soft tissues. Complex fractures typically include bicondylar fractures, metaphyseal-diaphyseal dissociations, and fracture-dislocation patterns.

J. Siegel, MD (✉)
Department of Orthopaedics,
UMass Memorial Medical Center,
55 Lake Avenue North, Worcester,
MA 01655, USA
e-mail: yoda5052@aol.com

P. Tornetta III, MD
Department of Orthopaedic Surgery,
Boston University Medical Center, Boston, MA, USA

6.2 Epidemiology

Complex tibial plateau fractures occur in two major groups of patients. The high-energy injuries typically present in the younger population and are more common in males than females. The lower-energy fractures, which are not necessarily less complex fractures, frequently occur in the older population, commonly females, and are often thought of as insufficiency fractures.

6.3 Traumatic Mechanism

High-energy fractures are often the result of motor vehicle crashes, falls from height, or pedestrian-struck injuries. These fractures are typically associated with more severe soft tissue damage and have a higher rate of neurovascular injuries, compartment syndrome, and open fractures than their lower energy counterparts. Lower-energy fractures result commonly

© Springer International Publishing Switzerland 2016
F. Castoldi, D.E. Bonasia (eds.), *Fractures Around the Knee*, Fracture Management Joint by Joint,
DOI 10.1007/978-3-319-28806-2_6

after simple falls in patients with osteopenic bone.

The magnitude, type, and direction of the force that injures the knee dictate the fracture pattern. Direct valgus force placed on the knee can result in the more simple plateau fracture patterns. Axial load is likely the primary force for the complex patterns with any associated valgus moment contributing to lateral impaction. Medial fractures and fracture-dislocations result from shearing forces often thought to occur when the knee is flexed, in varus, and then internally rotated. Bumper injuries from direct impact to the proximal tibia can result in separation of the condyles from the shaft and then extension into the joint. Although the articular component of these patterns may be simple, the soft tissue injury may be more severe.

6.4 Clinical Examination

Given the high rate of associated injuries, all patients who present with complex tibial plateau fractures should be examined for other associated orthopedic injuries. The mechanism of injury will assist with the clinical concerns regarding other injuries as well as the soft tissue injury about the knee and leg. Open wounds and fracture blisters affect the timing of surgical interventions and sometimes the surgical approach. The distal neurovascular examination must be meticulous despite often being difficult to obtain. A careful initial evaluation for tense compartments, pain with passive stretch, or altered distal pulses should be followed by repeat examinations in patients with fracture patterns associated with neurovascular injury or compartment syndrome [1]. Patients who require spanning external fixation must continue to be monitored for compartment syndrome after length is restored to the fracture as this may increase compartment pressures. Coronal plane instability is less subtle with complex fractures as these often require temporary external fixation to provide enough stability to allow for soft tissue healing and fracture reduction prior to definitive treatment.

6.5 Imaging and Preoperative Work-Up

To fully radiographically evaluate patients with high-energy bicondylar fractures, the principles of the joint above and the joint below should be followed. Additionally, femur films are especially necessary if a spanning external fixator is going to be used. At the minimum, orthogonal knee and tibia radiographs are required. Medial and lateral obliques and 10° caudal joint view plain films may obviate the need for a CT scan. In complex fractures or those in which further imaging is needed to define the fracture lines or the joint involvement for adequate preoperative planning, a CT scan should be obtained. Traction images obtained after spanning external fixation are typically more helpful in defining the pathoanatomy and are preferred by most surgeons. Therefore, if the initial images reveal a shortened or dislocated fracture, it is beneficial to wait until after a spanning external fixator is on to perform the advanced imaging studies.

6.6 Classification

Classically tibial plateau fractures are described with words describing the fracture lines and pattern. This is a useful practice since the fracture pattern dictates the treatment plan and these terms are well recognized by most surgeons. A commonly recognized and perhaps most widely used system that employs this technique is the Schatzker classification [2]. Although generally accepted as useful for the first three fracture types, problems exist when trying to classify fractures as type 4, 5, or 6. Medial fractures are considered type 4; however, there are several patterns of medial fractures and these cannot be delineated by Schatzker [3]. In particular, the "total condylar fracture-dislocation" pattern that leaves a portion of the lateral joint intact with the medial condyle and attached tibia dislocated is frequently misclassified as a Schatzker type 4, despite this pattern not appearing in the descriptive series. Type 5 fractures were originally described as medial and lateral condyle fractures with the intercondylar spines left intact, a pattern that rarely, if ever, can actually occur. More commonly, the medial condyle is a partial injury and the fracture should be classified as a variant of a fracture-dislocation. Type 6 fractures indicate metadiaphyseal dissociation and an articular component. Given the difficulty with the description of a type 5, many fractures are classified as type 6 because both condyles are fractured; however the metaphysis is not fractured from the diaphysis.

The OTA/AO alphanumeric system, commonly used for research purposes, is easily applied in this area of the body. A-type fractures are nonarticular and therefore technically not tibial plateau fractures. The partial B-type fractures can occur medially or laterally and are further characterized as simple split, articular depression, or split depression. The complete articular C-type fractures are further described based on level of complexity accounting for comminution of the joint or metaphysis. The fracture-dislocation pattern is not specifically described in this system either.

Given these issues with classifying tibial plateau fractures, most surgeons simply rely on describing the pattern, the fracture fragments, the presence of dislocation, and the level of comminution at the joint and the metaphysis. Familiarity with the classifications allows accurate use of the descriptive terminology and ultimately effective communication. This practice allows for the selection of surgical approaches and fixation methods.

6.7   Indications

The treatment goals in caring for patients with tibial plateau fractures are to restore alignment and to avoid complications. The protective nature of the meniscus makes the articular surface of the proximal tibia relatively resistant to posttraumatic arthrosis [4, 5]. Therefore understanding who needs surgical management is important as a few millimeters of step-off at the joint is not automatically a surgical indication as it can be for more constrained joints [6].

The difficulty in surgical decision-making for complex proximal tibia fractures lies in determining the optimal way to reduce and stabilize the fracture and less in indicating the patient for surgery. Unstable fractures in the coronal and/or sagittal planes and significant metaphyseal malalignment are reliable indications. This includes fracture-dislocations, metadiaphyseal dissociations, and bicondylar fractures. Medical comorbidities may make a patient with one of these injuries a nonsurgical candidate. Additionally, significant soft tissue injury may limit a surgeon's operative plan, but the unstable nature of the injury must still be addressed.

6.8   Timing of Surgical Treatment

Optimally, tibial plateau fractures should be fixed within 3 weeks of the injury due to ease of reduction. Low-energy fractures often present with minimal soft tissue injury and can safely be internally stabilized at any time in the first few weeks. It is the high-energy fractures that require sound decision-making and caution. Any patient who presents with an unstable, malaligned, or dislocated proximal tibia fracture and a concerning soft tissue envelope, staged fixation should be used. A knee spanning external fixation can be applied to restore length and alignment to the limb and allow for the soft tissues to heal. This often will take 10 days to 3 weeks to allow for swelling to subside and/or fracture blisters to resolve and epithelialize. The foot should not be included in the frame unless continuous compartment pressures are being monitored so that ankle motion and passive stretch can be tested. Once skin wrinkles are present in the areas of the skin incisions, it is typically safe to proceed.

6.9   Surgical Techniques

Choosing the appropriate surgical approach is the next step in successful management. Evaluating the radiographs and CT scan will determine the

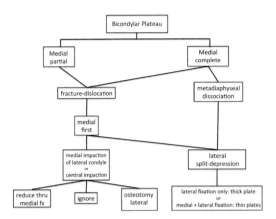

Fig. 6.1 Decision-making algorithm for bicondylar tibial plateau fractures and fracture-dislocations

optimal approach. Confirming that the soft tissue envelope in these areas is amenable to an incision is imperative. Typically the surgeon's initial decision is whether the fracture patterns warrant both medial and lateral fixation or simply unicondylar plating. The first key element in this decision is whether the medial condyle is complete or partial and whether there is a fracture-dislocation (Fig. 6.1).

If the medial condyle is a partial injury, then it is likely a fracture-dislocation pattern and the joint must be built from the medial side first, necessitating medial fixation. Similarly, if the medial condyle is complete, but there is a dislocation of the lateral side, medial fixation is required as this is a fracture-dislocation pattern. The only case in which isolated lateral fixation is reasonable is in a bicondylar fracture in which the medial side is complete and there is no dislocation present.

6.9.1   Lateral-Only Fixation

Some bicondylar fractures and metadiaphyseal fractures can be successfully treated with stiff, lateral fixed-angle plating only. The key to preventing fixation failure and varus collapse is the anatomy of the fracture on the medial side. If the fracture has a large medial condyle segment and cortical contact along the main medial fracture line (Fig. 6.2a), then stable fixation can be achieved with fracture reduction and a lateral

locked plate. In this example, the patient has a large medial condyle fracture and metadiaphyseal disassociation (Fig. 6.2b, c). The surgical plan was for an anterolateral approach only. The anterolateral incision was carried over the knee. The authors prefer a straight incision lateral to the tubercle instead of a hockey stick or a lazy S incision. The IT band and anterior compartment fascia are divided in line with the skin incision and the anterior compartment musculature is elevated off the proximal tibia. A submeniscal arthrotomy is performed and the lateral meniscus is identified, tagged, and inspected for tears. In this patient, the lateral meniscus was torn and found in the depressed segment. It was reduced to its native location and later would be repaired tying it down through the IT band. Elevation of the meniscus allows for visualization of the joint surface. The anterolateral fracture fragment is booked open. The metadiaphyseal component of the fracture is reduced first and held with percutaneously placed clamps and then lag screws (Fig. 6.2d, e). Then the joint surface is elevated and held reduced with Kirschner wires (K-wires). Allograft is packed into the defect to support the reduced joint. The cortical anterolateral fragment is reduced into its fracture bed and held reduced with bone holding forceps and K-wires. A lateral locked plate was slid submuscularly. Bicortical screws were placed in the shaft and locked screws were placed in the metaphysis (Fig. 6.2f, g). The medial column is aligned and together with the fixed-angle device allowed the patient to unite without varus collapse.

6.9.2   Medial and Lateral Fixation

Some bicondylar fractures include a large medial fragment in which the joint is otherwise intact and a more traditional lateral cortical disruption with joint impaction (Fig. 6.3a–c). An alternative approach to using a stiff lateral plate only, which may result in prominent hardware that is either painful later or difficult to cover, is to dual plate through two incisions with thinner, more flexible implants. Dual plating previously was associated with soft tissue complications, but most of those issues were done through a single incision [7]. Using a more soft tissue-friendly approach and thinner plates is another option to provide adequate fixation (Fig. 6.3d, e). Dual plating is almost always an option and many surgeons have moved completely away from thick lateral plates to avoid hardware irritation. The use of a thin medial plate to restore axial support transforms a type C injury to a type B partial articular injury and allows thin plating laterally. Medial and posteromedial plates can be easily placed though a small incision with minimal soft tissue

disruption, which makes this method attractive. The only contraindication is a comminuted metaphysis although a longer plate can be slid percutaneously down the tibia shaft to span these areas.

6.9.3 Posteromedial and Lateral Fixation

Most fracture-dislocation bicondylar fractures are associated with a posteromedial fragment

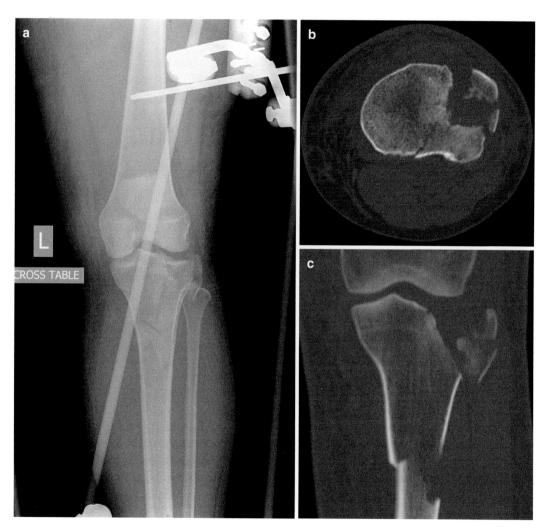

Fig. 6.2 Bicondylar metadiaphyseal tibial plateau fracture in a temporizing knee spanning external fixator (**a**) with CT scan cuts better defining the fractures (**b**, **c**). The patient underwent ORIF first by clamping the medial segment (**d**), stabilizing with lag screws and then reducing the lateral joint and holding with K-wires and then raft screws (**e**). Definitive internal fixation with a rigid lateral locking plate (**f**, **g**)

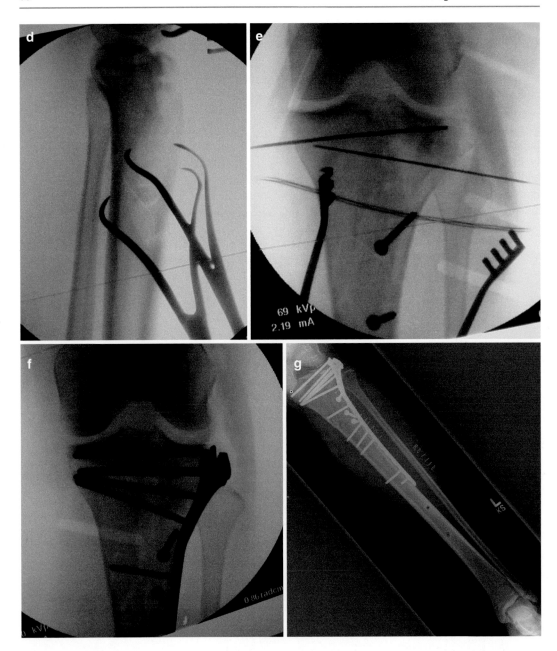

Fig. 6.2 (continued)

(Fig. 6.4a, b). These fragments are typically too small, too short, and/or too posterior to be captured by the screws from a lateral locking plate. Additionally, the shearing forces on that area of the plateau cannot be adequately neutralized with lateral-only fixation, and these patterns fail into varus (Fig. 6.5). Therefore, posteromedial antiglide plating is necessary to maintain alignment of the tibia and a reduction of the dislocation. The authors prefer to position the patient supine on a bump under the uninjured hip but prone positioning can also be used. The benefit of supine positioning is that the surgeon can simultaneously work both medially and laterally if necessary. An incision is made over the posteromedial border of the proximal tibia, anterior to the medial

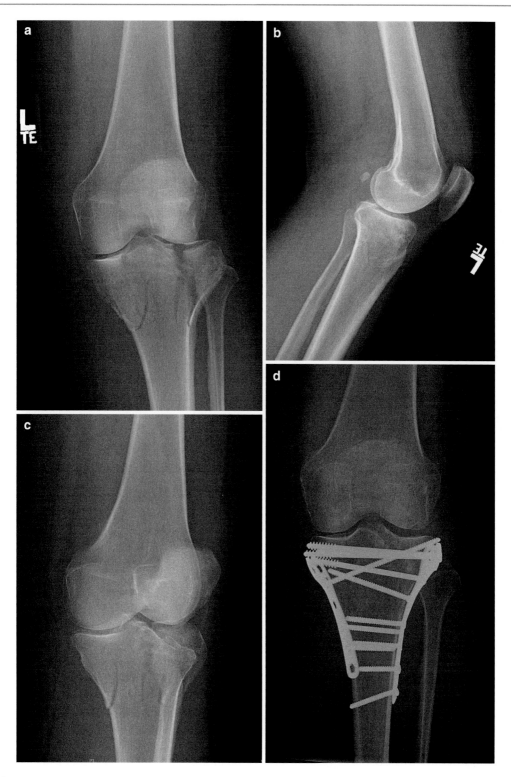

Fig. 6.3 Anteroposterior, lateral, external rotation oblique radiographs of a bicondylar fracture with a large medial segment but no metadiaphyseal dissociation (**a–c**). Soft tissue-friendly, thin, flexible plates were placed through two incisions to stabilize the fracture (**d, e**)

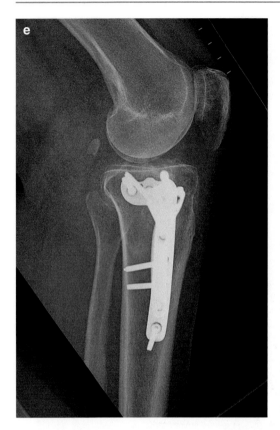

Fig. 6.3 (continued)

gastrocnemius muscle belly. The saphenous nerve and vein are protected during subcutaneous dissection. The deep interval is between the medial head of the gastrocnemius and the posterior border of the pes anserinus tendons. The posteromedial fracture fragment is often found in this interval. However, the fracture may interrupt the pes insertion, and in that situation, the dissection can be subperiosteal at the level of the fracture site with anterior and posterior elevation of the pes in both directions. This can be done with impunity.

After mobilizing and debriding any soft tissues and hematoma from the fracture, this fracture is reduced. If the injury is a fracture-dislocation and significantly displaced, the fracture can be difficult to reduce. A large periarticular reduction clamp can be placed medially through a poke hole onto the medial femoral condyle and laterally onto the lateral plateau to reduce the dislocated lateral joint and assist with overall alignment (Fig. 6.4c) [8]. Then an anterior-to-posterior Weber pointed bone tenaculum (the anterior tine typically placed through a poke hole anteriorly) will complete the anatomic reduction (Fig. 6.4d). Fluoroscopy is often necessary to confirm that the medial joint is reduced as the very common anteromedial fragment is often tilted and must be reduced before the posteromedial plate is applied. The reduction can be directly visualized at the articular surface by extending the incision a small amount proximally allowing for a small submeniscal release at the fracture site. This can be quite helpful if even the oblique fluoroscopy images do not show the joint well. While working on the medial side, always take care not to interfere with any future necessary work needed on the lateral side.

Lateral fixation in these types of bicondylar fractures is determined by the lateral pathology and should be individualized. In patients whose fractures require dual plating, thin implants can be used laterally and are easily covered during the soft tissue closure (Fig. 6.4e, f). The pathoanatomy is typically similar as described above. In some cases, the lateral cortex is not violated but the lateral joint is depressed. The surgeon must decide if the joint injury is severe enough to create instability and should be reduced and then how this area can be accessed. In the majority of cases, once the medial side is reduced and fixed, the lateral side is addressed as a standard lateral split depression fracture.

The one notable exception to this is the medial fracture-dislocation with impaction on the lateral side. This is a particular pattern as the lateral joint injury is medial from the lateral escape of the joint impinging the medial tibial surface on the femoral condyle as opposed to the typical lateral or central impaction seen with valgus injuries. An example of this is seen in Fig. 6.6a–d. Access to the central portion of the lateral joint may be limited as the lateral cortex may not be fractured. Additionally, as the impaction is located more medially, it is also less important to the survivorship of the joint which is peripherally loaded. In this situation, the lateral articular fragment may often be reduced from the medial side through the fracture site. In this case, it was pinned tem-

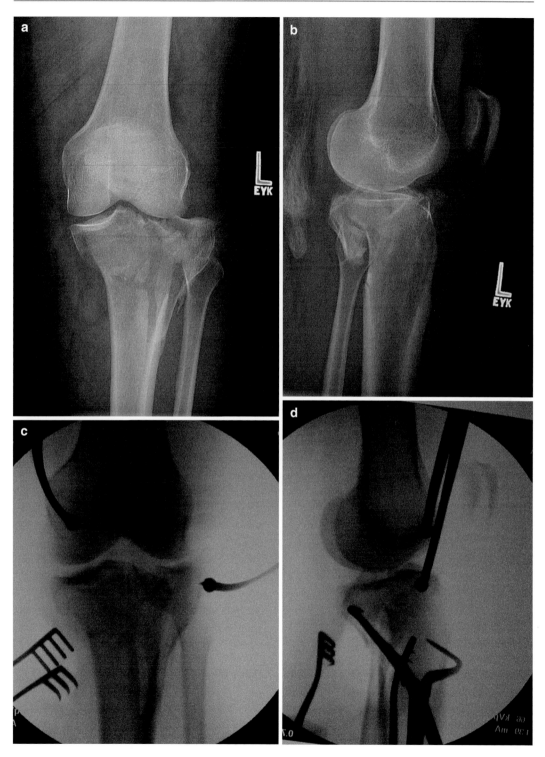

Fig. 6.4 Bicondylar fracture-dislocation plain radiographs showing the large posteromedial fragment, the lateral joint impaction, and the dislocated lateral joint (**a, b**). Intraoperative fluoroscopic image of a percutaneously placed large reduction forceps used to reduce the dislocation (**c**). Then a Weber clamp is placed to reduce the posteromedial fragment (**d**). The injury is stabilized with a posteromedial antiglide plate and a lateral buttress plate (**e, f**)

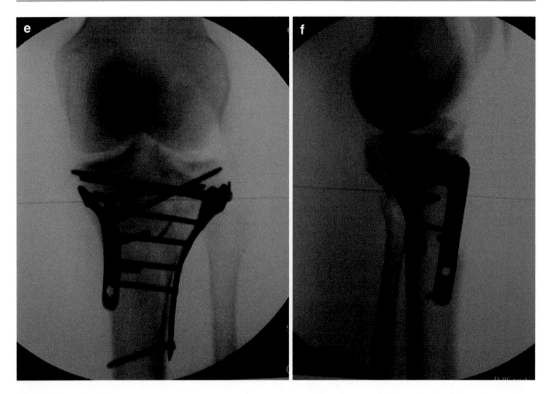

Fig. 6.4 (continued)

porarily with K-wires and then stabilized with a screw placed medially through the antiglide plate for the medial fracture. An additional percutaneous lag screw from the lateral side was later added.

6.10   Postoperative Regimen

After surgery, the patients are admitted to the hospital in order to be observed for development of compartment syndrome. Deep venous thrombosis prophylaxis is started the day after surgery. Passive range of motion is started immediately if there is no concern for the soft tissues. Since avoiding complications is paramount to a successful outcome and the soft tissue envelope can be unforgiving after a severe injury and surgery, if there are any concerns for the wound, the authors will immobilize the knee in full extension. The authors prefer full knee extension as opposed to 30° of flexion to avoid any possibility of losing terminal knee extension, which is more

difficult to regain later than knee flexion. Typically at 2–3 weeks postoperatively, the wound is healed and knee range of motion therapy is begun in a hinged brace. Given that most of these injuries are unstable in the coronal plane, the authors prefer a hinged brace to protect the repair.

Patients are maintained non-weight bearing for 12 weeks. With radiographic evidence of healing at that point, patients are allowed to advance their weight bearing as tolerated and can begin strengthening exercises. The brace is also discontinued at this point. Impact activities are limited until the patient has regained strength and conditioning in the extremity.

6.11   Complications

Avoiding complications is paramount to good outcomes in the treatment of severe tibial plateau fractures. Although recognizing the significance of the soft tissue injury has led to staged fixation,

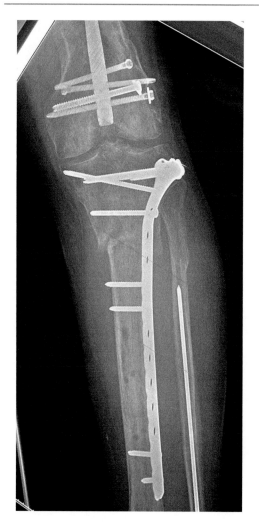

Fig. 6.5 Varus collapse of a metadiaphyseal fracture fixed with a rigid laterally based locking plate

treatment. Deformity correction must be included in the surgical planning. In a small series, union was achieved in four of five patients with 120° of knee motion but arthrosis is common [14]. Malunion is more common and likely contributes to arthrosis due to the alteration of joint contact forces.

Knee stiffness is often discussed but less common than expected despite temporizing knee joint spanning external fixation with even 6 weeks of knee spanning external fixation reported to have satisfactory motion outcomes [15]. Egol reported final knee range of motion of 1–106° after a staged protocol [12]. At 1-year follow-up, Rademakers reported an average range of motion of 130° (range 10–145°) [16].

Given the subcutaneous nature of the bone proximally, the triangular shape of the tibia, the thicker design of locking plates, and attempts to minimize surgical dissection, prominent hardware is common. Removal of the hardware can also result in unanticipated issues with crossthreading, stripped screw heads, and cold welding. The incidence and severity of these problems are unknown but are worth considering when deciding between a thicker, rigid plate and two incisions.

6.12 Results

The protective nature of the meniscus makes the articular surface of the proximal tibia relatively resistant to posttraumatic arthrosis [4, 5]. Nonetheless, the goals of surgery are to restore articular congruity and maintain alignment. Controversy exists as to which of these elements is more important. Outcome studies are varied and difficult to compare since many different knee scores are used and numerous secondary outcome measures are reported.

Bicondylar fractures with medial tilt and medial condyle fractures had worse outcomes in one study, with varus malalignment less tolerated than valgus [17]. The same authors reported that meniscectomy and malalignment correlated with arthrosis but articular step-off did not. Rademakers reported 31 % of his patients developed arthritis,

two incisions for dual plating, and careful handling of the soft tissues, the deep infection rates are still reported as 8.4–22 % [9–13]. Despite smaller incisions and minimally invasive techniques, deep infections are still difficult to resolve and require formal irrigation and debridement in the operating room, wounds left open to heal by secondary intentions, and hopes of infection suppression until the bone heals. Delaying hardware removal until after union is not always possible if the infection is aggressive. Tissue defects may require flap coverage, bony resection, and ultimately amputation.

Nonunion after tibial plateau fracture is rare. Infection must be excluded prior to attempts at

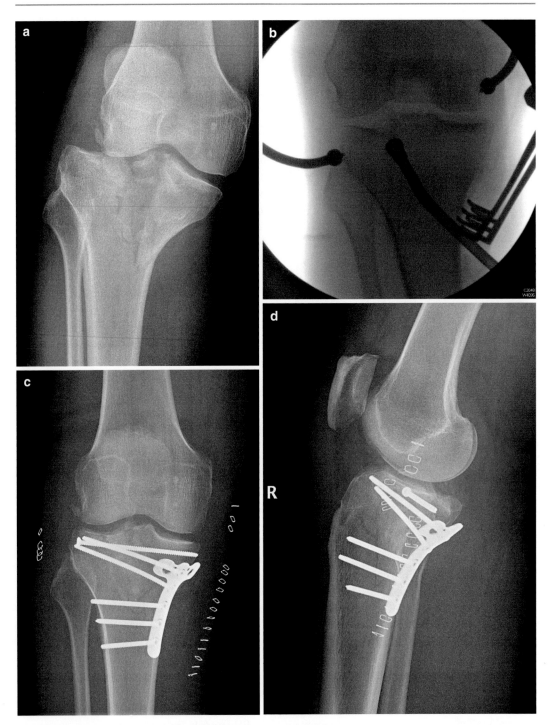

Fig. 6.6 Bicondylar fracture-dislocation in which the lateral cortex is intact but the medial portion of the lateral joint is depressed (**a**). The dislocation was reduced with a percutaneously placed clamp and the lateral joint surface was elevated through the medial fracture line (**b**). The medial side was stabilized with a posteromedial plate and the lateral joint was supported with medial and lateral raft screws (**c**, **d**)

which was well tolerated in 64 % at an average follow-up of 14 years. Patients with malalignment of more than 5° were more likely to develop arthritis than those with an anatomically aligned knee axis [16].

References

1. Stark E, Stucken C, Trainer G, Tornetta P (2009) Compartment syndrome in Schatzker type VI plateau fractures and medial condylar fracture-dislocations treated with temporary external fixation. J Orthop Trauma 23(7):502–506
2. Schatzker J, McBroom R, Bruce D (1979) The tibial plateau fracture. The Toronto experience 1968–1975. Clin Orthop Rel Res (138):94–104
3. Bhattacharyya T, McCarty L, Harris M (2005) The posterior shearing tibial plateau fracture: treatment and results via a posterior approach. J Orthop Trauma 19(5):305–310
4. Weiss N, Parvizi J, Trousdale R, Bryce R, Lewallen D (2003) Total knee arthroplasty in patients with a prior fracture of the tibial plateau. J Bone Joint Surg Am 85(2):218–221
5. Marsh J, Buckwalter J, Gelberman R, Dirschl D, Olson S, Brown T et al (2002) Articular fractures: does an anatomic reduction really change the result? J Bone Joint Surg Am 84(7):1259–1271
6. Rasmussen P (1973) Tibial condylar fractures. Impairment of knee joint stability as an indication for surgical treatment. J Bone Joint Surg Am 55(7):1331–1350
7. Young M, Barrack R (1994) Complications of internal fixation of tibial plateau fractures. Orthop Rev 23(2):149–154
8. Sibai T, Ricci W, Tornetta P (2015) Tibial plateau fracture subluxation: an effective intraoperative technique for the reduction of knee joint subluxation and associated medial tibial condyle fragments. Tech Orthop. epub
9. Barei D, Nork S, Mills W, Henley M, Benirschke S (2004) Complications associated with internal fixation of high-energy bicondylar tibial plateau fractures utilizing a two-incision technique. J Orthop Trauma 18(10):649–657
10. Canadian Orthopaedic Trauma Society (2006) Open reduction and internal fixation compared with circular fixator application for bicondylar tibial plateau fractures. Results of a multicenter, prospective, randomized clinical trial. J Bone Joint Surg Am 88(12):2613–2623
11. Shah S, Karunakar M (2007) Early wound complications after operative treatment of high energy tibial plateau fractures through two incisions. Bull NYU Hosp Jt Dis 65(2):115–119
12. Egol K, Tejwani N, Capla E, Wolinsky P, Koval K (2005) Staged management of high-energy proximal tibia fractures (OTA types 41): the results of a prospective, standardized protocol. J Orthop Trauma 19(7):448–455
13. Phisikul P, McKinley T, Nepola J, Marsh J (2007) Complications of locking plate fixation in complex proximal tibia injuries. J Orthop Trauma 21(2):83–91
14. Toro-Arbelaez J, Gardner M, Shindle M, Cabas J, Lorich D, Helfet D (2007) Open reduction and internal fixation of intraarticular tibial plateau nonunions. Injury 38(3):378–383
15. Marsh J, Smith S, Do T (1995) External fixation and limited internal fixation for complex fractures of the tibial plateau. J Bone Joint Surg Am 77(5):661–673
16. Rademakers M, Kerkhoffs G, Sierevelt I, Raaymakers E, Marti R (2007) Operative treatment of 109 tibial plateau fractures: five- to 27-year follow-up results. J Orthop Trauma 21(1):5–10
17. Honkonen S, Jarvinen M (1992) Classification of fractures of the tibial condyles. J Bone Joint Surg Br 74(6):840–847

Primary Total Knee Arthroplasty (TKA) in Tibial Plateau Fractures

7

Federica Rosso, Davide Blonna,
Antonio Marmotti, Gianluca Collo,
and Roberto Rossi

Abstract

Fifty percent of tibial plateau fractures occur in adult older than 50 years old, with 8–24 % of those occurring in elderly patients. The gold standard treatment for these fractures in young patients is open reduction and internal fixation (ORIF). However, because of poor bone quality, soft tissue impairment, and complications related to immobilization, ORIF in the elderly are associated to a high complication rate. For this reason, some authors proposed early total knee arthroplasty (TKA) to treat tibial plateau fractures in elderly patients affected by prior osteoarthritis. Surgeons approaching this surgery should be aware that the outcomes are inferior compared to elective TKA. Furthermore, the complication rate following TKA in tibial plateau fractures are more similar to revision TKA than primary TKA. For these reasons, early arthroplasty in proximal tibial fractures should be reserved to elderly patients affected by prior osteoarthritis, who do not comply with the restricted weight-bearing postoperative protocol in order to avoid further surgery. There are few reports on literature reporting on the outcomes of early TKA in tibial plateau fractures, with small records and short follow-up. However, the authors agree in defining this procedure as a valid option in these patients.

This chapter reviewed indications, surgical techniques, and outcomes of TKA to treat acute tibial plateau fracture.

F. Rosso (✉) • D. Blonna • A. Marmotti
AO Mauriziano Umberto I,
SCDU Ortopedia e Traumatologia,
Largo Turati 62, Torino 10128, Italy
e-mail: federica.rosso@yahoo.it

G. Collo
Dipartimento di Ortopedia Traumatologia
e Riabilitazione, AO Città della Salute e della Scienza,
Via Zuretti 29, Torino 10126, Italy

R. Rossi
AO Mauriziano Umberto I,
SCDU Ortopedia e Traumatologia,
Largo Turati 62, Torino 10128, Italy

Dipartimento di Scienze Chirurgiche,
Università degli Studi di Torino,
Via Po 8, Torino 10100, Italy

© Springer International Publishing Switzerland 2016
F. Castoldi, D.E. Bonasia (eds.), *Fractures Around the Knee*, Fracture Management Joint by Joint,
DOI 10.1007/978-3-319-28806-2_7

Keywords
Knee • Tibial plateau • Fracture • Post-traumatic • Arthritis • Arthroplasty
Outcomes • Elderly

7.1   Introduction

The annual incidence of tibial plateau fracture is 13.3 per 100,000 adult patients. Approximately half of these fractures occur in patient older than 50 years old, with 8–24 % occurring in the elderly population [6]. Open reduction and internal fixation (ORIF) is often the treatment of choice in young patients [10]. Some authors underlined the difficulties to obtain a stable fixation, as well as the higher risk of losing reduction in elderly patients treated with ORIF [8]. Furthermore there is a concern regarding the risk of wound healing consequent to the soft tissue stripping needed for ORIF as well as the poor compliance to the restriction in weight-bearing often necessary after fracture fixation [20]. Some authors described an unacceptable failure rate (79 %) and unsatisfactory results for ORIF in elderly patients [1]. For these reasons there is still a concern about treating tibial plateau fractures in elderly patients using ORIF [4].

The main complications reported in the literature for ORIF in tibial plateau fractures are loss of correction, post-traumatic arthritis requiring subsequent total knee arthroplasty (TKA), malunion or nonunion, stiffness, and medical comorbidities secondary to the immobilization. Secondary TKA in patients with previous tibial plateau fracture may be challenging because of ligament imbalance, extensor mechanism scars, patellar maltracking, and lower limb deformity. Different authors reported higher complication and reoperation rates in patients who underwent secondary TKA with a prior tibial plateau fracture compared with primary TKA [26, 27].

All these data, associated to the higher risk of complication derived from the immobilization in elderly, led several authors to propose TKA in the acute treatment of tibial plateau fractures in this population [3, 4, 9, 11, 12, 14, 24].

7.2   Indications

Total knee arthroplasty (TKA) may be an option in elderly patients with tibial plateau fractures and previous osteoarthritis. The main advantage of TKA compared to ORIF is the early mobilization, which can be fundamental in elderly patients. However, there is still a concern regarding mechanical failure, loosening, and periprosthetic fractures, so this treatment should be reserved to elderly sedentary patients [16]. A relative contraindication to primary TKA to treat tibial plateau fracture is the avulsion of the tibial tubercle, because of the high rate of nonunion that is really challenging to manage [4, 19].

In conclusion, surgeons should consider primary TKA in tibial plateau fractures for elderly sedentary patients, affected by preexisting arthritis, with difficulties to comply with restricted weight-bearing and with comminuted type C intra-articular fractures and in the patients where a second surgery is contraindicated [3] (Table 7.1).

Table 7.1 Summary of indication and contraindication to primary TKA in tibial plateau fractures

Indication	Relative contraindication
Elderly patients	Young patients
Preexisting osteoarthritis	Tibial tubercle avulsion
Comminuted type C intra-articular fractures	Extra-articular fractures
Patients in which is preferable to avoid: Immobilization (high complication risk) Secondary procedures	

7.3 Imaging and Preoperative Work-Up

Accurate preoperative planning is mandatory in TKA [18]. In acute trauma, the planning cannot be as accurate as in elective TKA, because there are no weight-bearing X-rays to evaluate the radiological alignment. Anteroposterior and lateral X-rays at rest are mandatory to evaluate the amount of femoral resection, posterior osteophytes together with patellar height, and tracking. Computed tomography (CT) scan is useful to classify the fracture morphology and to identify the amount of bone loss [5]. Furthermore, it is necessary to plan the steps of the surgery, as in ORIF. Figure 7.1 shows preoperative X-rays and CT scan of an 80-year-old female with tibial plateau fracture.

Clinical evaluation is fundamental. First of all, the soft tissue quality should be evaluated; primary TKA should not be performed if inadequate soft tissue covering is anticipated. Furthermore ligamentous stability should be checked, according with the fracture morphology, to decide the grade of constraint needed, and this should be planned preoperatively [3].

7.4 Implant Selection

The first problem the surgeon has to face approaching a primary TKA in proximal tibial plateau fracture is the grade of constraint to use. The minimum amount of constraint needed to achieve knee stability should be chosen, minimizing the risk of loosening. The same principles used in revision TKA can be applied to TKA in tibial plateau fracture [3, 4].

7.5 Surgical Technique

Surgical technique for TKA in tibial plateau fracture is a little bit different compared to elective TKA. Nevertheless, the basic principles normally used in elective TKA, such as gap balancing, are applicable also in these patients. For some crucial points, such as use of longer stem for the treatment of bone losses, the same principle used in revision TKA can be applied.

The surgeon should plan the incision accurately, to enable the addition of any internal fixation. A midline incision, as well as in elective

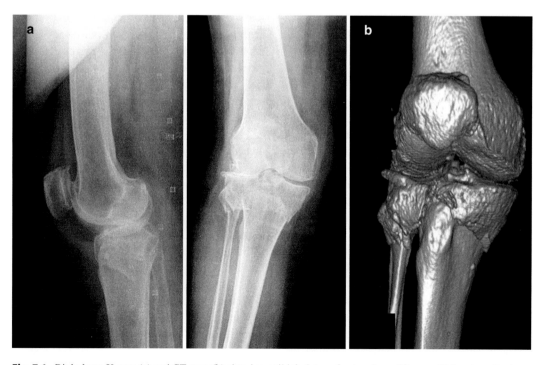

Fig. 7.1 Right knee X-rays (**a**) and CT scan (**b**) showing a tibial plateau fracture in an 80-year-old female patient

Fig. 7.2 Postoperative
X-rays (anteroposterior and
lateral views) of an 80-year-
old female with right tibial
plateau fracture treated with
rotating hinge TKA with
stems

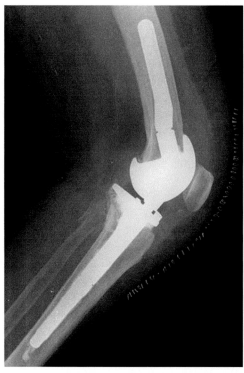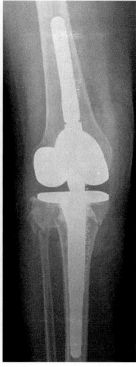

TKA, is often the best choice for this purpose [3, 4, 11]. The surgery continues with a medial para-patellar arthrotomy, to expose the joint; serious attention should be paid to the patellar tendon, to avoid avulsion. Once the joint is exposed, the fracture should be evaluated.

Surgeon can use the "three-step technique" introduced by Vince for revision TKA [25]. The first step is the restoration of the tibial platform, then the stabilization of the knee in flexion, with evaluation of femoral rotation and joint line height, and, lastly, the stabilization of the knee in extension. The joint line restoration and evaluation of component rotation, both on femoral and tibial side, can be more challenging compared to elective TKA, particularly in patients with major bone loss. Temporary fracture reduction and fixation using K-wires may be useful in identifying the standard anatomical landmarks to asses both component rotation and joint line height. Other landmarks, such as the tip of the fibula or the inferior pole of the patella, can be used, as well as in revision TKA [14, 25]. Once the anatomy is partially reestablished, the tibial cut can be performed, taking care to preserve as much bone as possible.

During the cuts, temporary fixation can be used to stabilize the fracture. Some authors suggested to use intramedullary alignment guide on both the femoral and tibial side, to simplify the conversion to stemmed implants that are often necessary in these patients [3, 4]. During restoration of the tibial platform, the authors have to face with bone loss and the need of stems. Different authors suggested using uncemented stems on the tibial side to obtain a diaphyseal fixation in case of bone defects. When the fracture extends over the metaphyseal-diaphyseal junction or in the diaphyseal portion of the tibia, some authors suggested using longer stem to bypass the fracture and obtain a kind of intramedullary fixation [9]. However, there is some agreement in literature in using longer tibial stems in type C intra-articular comminuted fracture involving the metaphyseal portion of the tibia and in associating higher constrained implants. In cases of simple split-depression fracture treated with TKA, a standard implant can be used [24]. Figure 7.2 shows the postoperative X-rays (anteroposterior and lateral view) of an 80-year-old female with tibial plateau fracture treated with stemmed rotating hinge TKA.

In approaching TKA for tibial plateau fractures in elderly, treatment of bone defects is often challenging. The same principles used for revision TKA should be applied. The bone defect should be first classified according to the Anderson Orthopaedic Research Institute (AORI) classification [7]. In this classification, the femur (F) and tibial (T) side are considered separately. Type 1 defects do not affect the metaphyseal portion and do not affect knee stability; in type 2 defects the metaphyseal bone is damaged and one condyle is involved. In type 3 defects the metaphyseal portion is reabsorbed with involvement of both the condyles. Different options are available to manage bone defects, including cement, cement with screw augmentation, modular metallic wedges, bone autograft or allograft, sleeves, cone-shape augments, and custom-made prostheses. In AORI type I defects, some authors suggested to fill bone loss (< than 5 mm in depth and width) using cement [17, 23]. In case of mild contained or uncontained defects >5 mm but <10 mm, cement with screws is indicated, to better distribute the load away from the joint line. Five or 6.5 mm screws should be placed 5–10 mm apart. Some authors suggested using bone graft when the cement mantle below the tibial plateau is >5 mm thick [17, 21]. In type 2 defects, cement is not sufficient to restore the platform. Impacted morcellized bone grafts are indicated in contained defects larger than 10 mm or uncontained defects <50 % of the tibial plateau, without involvement of the cortical bone [22]. Metal augments can be useful in treating these defects and are normally indicated in cases or more than 50 % of plateau involvement. However, these augments can manage bone defects only up to 20 mm in depth because of the loosening risk [15]. In type III defects, structural allografts are indicated for segmental defects smaller than 15 mm for the femur and greater than 20–45 mm for the tibia [2]. To fill these defects, also tantalum cones or metallic sleeves can be used [9].

The second step of the surgery is to restore the knee balance in flexion, choosing the right femoral component size and rotation and establishing the correct joint line height. The same rules of revision TKA should be applied to this step: bone loss should not be considered in order not to undersize the component. The contralateral knee may be useful to choose the component size and to avoid too large flexion gaps [25]. Some authors suggested avoiding femoral stems if possible, mostly in patients with ipsilateral hip arthroplasty, because of the increased risk of periprosthetic fractures [24]. To assess the femoral component rotation and the correct joint line height, different anatomic landmarks can be useful, such as the trans-epicondylar axis and epicondyle.

Once the component size and rotation are established, and the correct joint line is achieved, the third phase is to restore the knee stability in extension. The surgeon should remember to avoid increasing polyethylene thickness to stabilize the knee in extension, because of joint line alteration. Extension stability should be achieved distalizing the femoral component. The same principles described in the "three-step technique" for revision TKA can be applied also to TKA in tibial plateau fracture [25].

Bohm et al. suggested that fracture fragments must be stably fixed and protected with intramedullary stems to allow early weight-bearing. Furthermore, they proposed an algorithm to treat tibial plateau fracture using TKA based on Schatzker's classification. In Schatzker type III fractures, with depression of the lateral tibial plateau, the defects can be filled with cement if smaller than 1 cm or a cancellous bone graft if it is larger. In these cases, if there is good circumferential cortical bone stock, superficial prosthesis without stems can be used. In presence of uncontained bone defects, tibial augments and stems are mandatory to restore the metaphyseal support and to guarantee a stable fixation, in association with longer stems. In Schatzker types I, II, and IV, the authors suggested using intramedullary fixation, supplemented by internal fixation if the fragments are large enough. Finally Schatzker type V and VI involving both condyles, with or without metaphyseal extension, are the most demanding to manage, and the authors suggested a combination of tibial stems and plate fixation [4].

In the literature, there is still a debate on routine patellar replacement in elective TKA.

Table 7.2 Results of primary total knee arthroplasty (TKA) in tibial plateau fractures

Authors	Number of cases	Mean age (range)	Implants	Average follow-up	Outcomes
Nau et al. [12]	6 knees	79 years (range 70–90)	Five rotating hinged and one unconstrained implant	24.4 months	No loosening at follow-up. Two patients were free of pain and four patients reported mild or occasional pain. In five cases, the knee flexion ranged from 70° to 110°. All the patients used cane or walkers
Nourissat et al. [13]	4 knees	Over 75 years old	Constrained; long-stem, cemented tibial component when epiphysis reconstruction	2–7 years	Three knees graded as excellent. Bone healing in all the cases. No radiolucent lines
Vermeire et al. [24]	12 knees	73 years (range 53–81)	11 cemented posterior stabilized and 1 constrained condylar TKA with a stemmed tibial component bypassing the fracture area. Bone losses: cemented stems (2), graft impaction (5), augmentation (2). Seven cases of additional fixation	31 months	Nine patients with normal alignment and two with valgus one. The mean knee flexion was 115.9° (95–130°). The median final knee score was 78 points (range: 50–100) and the median function score 58 (range: 0–100). Seven patients were rated as excellent. No signs of loosening, no revision required
Parratte et al. [14]	26 knees (16 proximal tibial and 10 distal femoral fractures)	80.5 years (range 70–98)	21 postero-stabilized (9 standard implant and 12 revision endomedullary implants). Five rotating hinge prostheses	16.2 months	23 % immediate general complications and 15 % of local arthroplasty-related complications. The mean active extension deficit was 4.1°. The mean IKS knee score was 82 points. The function score was 54 point
Malviya et al. [11]	25 knees (15 proximal tibial and 10 distal femoral fractures)	80 years (range 67–92)	Depends on fracture morphology and surgeon preference	38.8 months	90 % of patients were satisfied. Mean Knee Society knee score was 90.2, Knee Society function score was 35.5, Oxford Knee Score was 39.5, and Short Form (SF)-36 physical function score was 37.3 and mental score 50.6
Kini et al. [9]	9 knees (Six lateral tibial plateau fractures and three diaphyseal fractures)	Not available	Five postero-stabilized implant, six cases of bony defect filled with cement and two cases with tantalum metaphyseal cone, all tibial stem (longer in diaphyseal fractures)	26 months	Average range of movement (ROM) was 114° (95–125°). Mean Knee Society score was 84. Out of nine cases, five were graded as excellent, three good, and one fair
Benazzo et al. [3]	6 knees	62 years (range 47–76 years)	Postero-stabilized and condylar-constrained implants	12 months	Mean postoperative clinical KSS was 84 (Range 50–100). Five patients were graded as good or excellent. No radiolucent lines

However, patellar replacement seems a reasonable option in TKA in tibial plateau fracture to reduce the risk of further surgeries [4].

7.6   Results

There are few reports in the literature regarding the outcomes of primary TKA in tibial plateau fractures. However, despite hip replacement is a well-accepted treatment for proximal femoral fractures, it is not for TKA in tibial plateau fractures [24].

Nau et al. were probably the first to report the outcomes of TKA in six patients with tibial plateau fractures. In five cases, a rotating hinge implant was used. The authors concluded about moderate functional outcomes, with an average flexion ranging from 70° to 110° [12].

One year later Nourissat described the results of four patients who underwent the same treatment, with three excellent outcomes. The authors concluded that TKA as a primary treatment for complex tibial plateau fractures in elderly is an acceptable option [13].

Vermiere et al. described one of the largest case series (12 patients). The authors reported good clinical outcomes in these patients and concluded that TKA is a suitable option for complex tibial plateau fractures in elderly patients affected by prior osteoarthritis [24].

Paratte et al. evaluated 26 patients from different centers in Europe. Ten patients were treated for distal femoral fractures, while the remaining for proximal tibial. The authors described 23 % of immediate general complications and 15 % of local knee-related complications. With these data they concluded that TKA is a suitable option for complex distal femoral or proximal tibial fracture in elderly patients, but the complication rate is higher compared to elective TKA and comparable to TKA in post-traumatic arthritis [14].

Other authors confirmed these results, concluding that, similarly to hip arthroplasty for proximal femoral fractures, primary TKA may be an option to treat proximal tibial fractures in elderly patients with osteoporosis and/or osteoarthritis [3, 11].

There is only one report on the role of navigation in this procedure. Kini et al. reported their results on nine patients (six affected by a lateral tibial plateau fractures and three by diaphyseal fractures) treated with primary navigated TKAs. The authors used a postero-stabilized implant in most of the tibial plateau fractures and reserved longer stem to the cases with diaphyseal involvement. In this study five patients out of nine were graded as excellent [9].

Table 7.2 shows summaries of these results.

Conclusion

ORIF is the gold standard treatment in proximal tibial fractures. However, ORIF may be challenging in elderly patients due to poor bone quality and ligamentous instability. Considering the good results achieved in hip arthroplasty following proximal femoral fractures, some authors proposed TKA to treat fractures around the knee, particularly proximal tibial fractures. This treatment may be reasonable in elderly patients affected by complex type C intra-articular proximal tibial fractures, due to poor bone quality and high complication rates following ORIF. There are few reports in the literature describing the results of early TKA in tibial plateau fractures, with small records and short follow-up. However, most of the authors concluded that this technique is a safe treatment, with good outcomes. However, outcomes are inferior to elective TKA and similar to TKA in post-traumatic arthritis.

In conclusion, TKA in tibial plateau fracture should be reserved to elderly patients affected by prior osteoarthritis. Surgeons should expect a higher complication rate, more similar to revision TKA than to primary TKA.

References

1. Ali AM, El-Shafie M, Willett KM (2002) Failure of fixation of tibial plateau fractures. J Orthop Trauma 16(5):323–329

2. Backstein D, Safir O, Gross A (2006) Management of bone loss: structural grafts in revision total knee arthroplasty. Clin Orthop Relat Res 446:104–112. doi:10.1097/01.blo.0000214426.52206.2c

3. Benazzo F, Rossi SM, Ghiara M, Zanardi A, Perticarini L, Combi A (2014) Total knee replacement in acute and chronic traumatic events. Injury 45(Suppl 6):S98–S104. doi:10.1016/j.injury.2014.10.031

4. Bohm ER, Tufescu TV, Marsh JP (2012) The operative management of osteoporotic fractures of the knee: to fix or replace? J Bone Joint Surg 94(9):1160–1169. doi:10.1302/0301-620X.94B9.28130

5. Brunner A, Horisberger M, Ulmar B, Hoffmann A, Babst R (2010) Classification systems for tibial plateau fractures; does computed tomography scanning improve their reliability? Injury 41(2):173–178. doi:10.1016/j.injury.2009.08.016

6. Court-Brown CM, Bugler KE, Clement ND, Duckworth AD, McQueen MM (2012) The epidemiology of open fractures in adults. A 15-year review. Injury 43(6):891–897. doi:10.1016/j.injury.2011.12.007

7. Engh GA, Ammeen DJ (1999) Bone loss with revision total knee arthroplasty: defect classification and alternatives for reconstruction. Instr Course Lect 48:167–175

8. Honkonen SE (1994) Indications for surgical treatment of tibial condyle fractures. Clin Orthop Relat Res 302:199–205

9. Kini SG, Sathappan SS (2013) Role of navigated total knee arthroplasty for acute tibial fractures in the elderly. Arch Orthop Trauma Surg 133(8):1149–1154. doi:10.1007/s00402-013-1792-8

10. Krupp RJ, Malkani AL, Roberts CS, Seligson D, Crawford CH, 3rd, Smith L (2009) Treatment of bicondylar tibia plateau fractures using locked plating versus external fixation. Orthopedics 32(8):559. doi:10.3928/01477447-20090624-11

11. Malviya A, Reed MR, Partington PF (2011) Acute primary total knee arthroplasty for peri-articular knee fractures in patients over 65 years of age. Injury 42(11):1368–1371. doi:10.1016/j.injury.2011.06.198

12. Nau T, Pflegerl E, Erhart J, Vecsei V (2003) Primary total knee arthroplasty for periarticular fractures. J Arthroplasty 18(8):968–971

13. Nourissat G, Hoffman E, Hemon C, Rillardon L, Guigui P, Sautet A (2006) Total knee arthroplasty for recent severe fracture of the proximal tibial epiphysis in the elderly subject. Rev Chir Orthop Reparatrice Appar Mot 92(3):242–247

14. Parratte S, Bonnevialle P, Pietu G, Saragaglia D, Cherrier B, Lafosse JM (2011) Primary total knee arthroplasty in the management of epiphyseal fracture around the knee. Orthop Traumatol Surg Res: OTSR 97(6 Suppl):S87–S94. doi:10.1016/j.otsr.2011.06.008

15. Patel JV, Masonis JL, Guerin J, Bourne RB, Rorabeck CH (2004) The fate of augments to treat type-2 bone defects in revision knee arthroplasty. J Bone Joint Surg 86(2):195–199

16. Ries MD (2012) Primary arthroplasty for management of osteoporotic fractures about the knee. Curr Osteoporos Rep 10(4):322–327. doi:10.1007/s11914-012-0122-3

17. Ritter MA, Keating EM, Faris PM (1993) Screw and cement fixation of large defects in total knee arthroplasty. A sequel. J Arthroplasty 8(1):63–65

18. Robbins GM, Masri BA, Garbuz DS, Duncan CP (2001) Preoperative planning to prevent instability in total knee arthroplasty. Orthop Clin North Am 32(4):611–626, viii

19. Saleh KJ, Sherman P, Katkin P, Windsor R, Haas S, Laskin R, Sculco T (2001) Total knee arthroplasty after open reduction and internal fixation of fractures of the tibial plateau: a minimum five-year follow-up study. J Bone Joint Surg Am 83-A(8):1144–1148

20. Scharf S, Christophidis N (1994) Fractures of the tibial plateau in the elderly as a cause of immobility. Aust N Z J Med 24(6):725–726

21. Scott RD (1995) Bone loss: prosthetic and augmentation method. Orthopedics 18(9):923–926

22. Suarez-Suarez MA, Murcia A, Maestro A (2002) Filling of segmental bone defects in revision knee arthroplasty using morsellized bone grafts contained within a metal mesh. Acta Orthop Belg 68(2):163–167

23. Toms AD, Barker RL, McClelland D, Chua L, Spencer-Jones R, Kuiper JH (2009) Repair of defects and containment in revision total knee replacement: a comparative biomechanical analysis. J Bone Joint Surg 91(2):271–277. doi:10.1302/0301-620X.91B2.21415

24. Vermeire J, Scheerlinck T (2010) Early primary total knee replacement for complex proximal tibia fractures in elderly and osteoarthritic patients. Acta Orthop Belg 76(6):785–793

25. Vince KG Oakes DA (2006) Three-step technique for revision total knee arthroplasty. In: Knee arthroplasty handbook. Springer, New York, pp 104–115

26. Weiss NG, Parvizi J, Hanssen AD, Trousdale RT, Lewallen DG (2003) Total knee arthroplasty in post-traumatic arthrosis of the knee. J Arthroplasty 18(3 Suppl 1):23–26. doi:10.1054/arth.2003.50068

27. Weiss NG, Parvizi J, Trousdale RT, Bryce RD, Lewallen DG (2003) Total knee arthroplasty in patients with a prior fracture of the tibial plateau. J Bone Joint Surg Am 85-A(2):218–221

Floating Knee

8

Qiugen Wang, Lei Cao, Jianhong Wu, Jian Lin, and Xiaoxi Ji

8.1 Epidemiology

Floating knee is the term applied to a flail knee joint segment resulting from fractures of the shaft or adjacent metaphysis of the ipsilateral femur and tibia [1] (Figs. 8.1 and 8.2).

Although the precise incidence of a floating knee is not known, it is a relatively uncommon injury. High-energy trauma is the main cause of this injury complex. The incidence seems more frequently in developing countries because of increased number of automobiles and motorcycles. Young male adults, especially in the age range of 20–30 years, make the largest proportion of this disease [2].

The high-energy trauma not only causes extensive comminution and displacement of the fracture but also leads to severe neurovascular injury and soft tissue damage. The stress from lateral or anteroposterior can cause disruption of ligamentous complex of the knee joint. In addition, associated life-threatening injuries to the head, chest, or abdomen take precedence over treatment of the fractures.

Q. Wang (✉) • L. Cao • J. Wu • J. Lin • X. Ji
Shanghai Trauma & Emergency Center,
Shanghai General Hospital,
Shanghai Jiao Tong University,
650 Xinsongjiang Road,
Shanghai 201600, China
e-mail: wangqiugen@163.com; caoleiseu@163.com;
wujianhong1978@163.com; linjian1981@126.com;
jixiaoxi87@163.com

Vascular damage is quite common due to the traction or the oppression of the bone block. Arterial lacerations occur in 30 % of the cases, mainly to the popliteal and posterior tibial arteries. The incidence of nerve dysfunction is approximately 10 %, and the most commonly affected nerve is the peroneal nerve, as a result of traction injury [3, 4].

The incidence of open fractures is very high, approaching 50–70 % at one or both fracture sites. The most common combination is a closed femoral fracture with an open tibial fracture. The medial tibial is located in the subcutaneous and therefore is easy to be exposed.

The incidence of knee ligament injuries is probably 30–40 % of the patients [5, 6]. Joint swelling and severe pain during physical examination make the diagnosis of ligamentous injuries very difficult. The relationship between the type of the fracture and which ligaments are involved is not clear. Associated trauma to the head, chest, abdomen, pelvis, and long bones of the contralateral extremity is common. The reported rate of such injuries may be as high as 89 % [7], underlining the high energy of the traumatic mechanism.

8.2 Traumatic Mechanism

High-velocity traffic accident is the most common mechanism of trauma (reported up to 97 %), followed by a fall from a height [8]; gunshot

Fig. 8.1 Fraser's classification

Type I   Type IIa   Type IIb   Type IIc

Type A: diaphyseal closed

Type C: epiphyseal and diaphyseal

Type B: metaphyseal and diaphyseal closed

Type D: one fracture open

Type E: two fracture open

Open →   ← Open

← Open

Fig. 8.2 Letts and Vincent classification

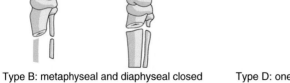
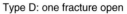
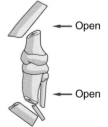

wounds and machine injury are relatively rare causes.

In motor vehicle collisions, the knees of the bikers/cyclists or the car occupants are stroked by strong and direct violence, and the knee joints lose continuity with both the femur and tibia. The isolated joints are unstable and "float," and some residual energy may hurt the hip, the acetabulum, or the ankle. Due to the high energy, multiple organ injuries and other bone fractures are common, which makes the injury more complicated and difficult to handle.

The floating knee is not common in children and is mainly caused when a child cyclist collides with a car. It is assumed that during the accident, the tibia and fibula are initially fractured by the bumper of the car, and then the femur is fractured by the front of the car, while head, chest, or abdomen injuries are due to the rolling on the hood and falling on the ground. Skin or soft tissue injuries may occur when the limb is compressed by the wheels [9].

Floating knee injury caused by firearm is rare and has some specific features: (1) bone injury is serious and complex, the high energy transferred from the projectiles and many pieces from different directions and angles hit the same location of the limb, and can cause severe open comminuted fractures and multi-segmental and severely displaced fractures; (2) soft tissue damage is serious and wound contamination is common; and (3) the high incidence of hemodynamic shock, open fractures, severe soft tissue damage, and associated injuries commonly result in high incidence of shock.

8.3 Clinical Examination

The floating knee is often a result of high-energy trauma and may be associated with life-threatening injuries. Fracture patterns are often complex with serious injuries of the soft tissues. The affected limb is always swollen and deformity is evident. After the first examination, resuscitation (if necessary), and splinting of the affected limb, the patient should be thoroughly examined a second time from head to toe to exclude associated fractures. Besides bone and soft tissue injuries, the patients' general condition should be monitored carefully. Vascular assessment of the affected limb is of utmost importance in detecting any vascular injury by assessing the peripheral pulses by palpation or Doppler.

8.4 Imaging and Preoperative Work-Up

8.4.1 Imaging

The long-leg x-rays of the affected limb are needed in the primary examination. The radiography of the unaffected side is helpful for the preparation of the preoperative plan. CT scan is also helpful to determine the detail of the fracture pattern in some severely comminuted fractures.

The incidence of knee ligament injuries can be as high as 53 % in floating knee patients [3, 5]. Knee ligamentous and meniscal injuries are mostly not visible in plain radiographs taken in the emergency department and are likely to be overlooked by clinicians. So, when the patients' general conditions are stable, MRI of the affected knee is recommended.

Besides this, radiographs of the chest, pelvis, affected lower limb including all its joints, and other suspected bony injuries are also needed.

If vascular injury is suspected, ultrasound and angiography are needed. Evaluation of abdominal injuries should be performed by clinical assessment and ultrasound. If there is suspicion of intra-abdominal or cerebral injury, an urgent CT scan is indicated.

8.4.2 Preoperative Work-Up

The treatment of floating knee should initially manage the general conditions of the patients, solving the associated life-threatening injuries and preventing shock and fat embolism. Saving the life is the priority, replenishing the blood volume and treating the fat embolism syndrome. When the general condition is stable, the treatment of fracture should be considered: (1) In open fractures, initial wound toilet, tetanus immunization, and antibiotic therapy should be initiated. (2) The surgical timing depends on the general condition of the patients, and the severity of the associated injury, the condition of the local soft tissue and blood and nerve injury, the experiences and surgical techniques of the surgical team, and the condition of the hospital equipments are also important. When encountered in the elderly, the diminished physiologic reserve and preexisting comorbidities may result in a higher rate of complication and mortality than in young patients. The principle here is to manage the patient's comorbidities (cardiorespiratory, renal, etc.) until the patient is fit to undergo surgery [10, 11]. (3) Like some other intra-articular fractures, there is no evidence that these fractures need to be fixed definitively in emergency; however, temporary external fixation of the fracture is advised until the general and local conditions of the patient are stable. This time can be useful to correctly plan the surgery. (4) The timing of vascular repair and bone stabilization is debated. McHenry et al. [12] found no iatrogenic disruption of the vascular repair when bone stabilization followed vascular repair. The general consensus is that bone stabilization should precede vascular repair in unstable fractures, while in stable fractures, vascular repair should be done first to avoid prolonged ischemia to the limb. (5) If significant abdominal injuries are detected, these take priority over surgical stabilization of the fractures.

8.5   Classification

1. *Blake and Mcbryde*:
   "True" or type I injury: pure diaphyseal fracture of the femur and tibia
   "Variant" or type II: fracture extends into the knee, hip, or ankle joint [1].

2. *Fraser's classification*:
   Most commonly used, according to knee involvement
   Type I: extra-articular fractures of femur and tibia
   Type II: divided into three groups:
   IIa: fractures of femoral shaft and tibial plateau
   IIb: fractures of distal femur and shaft of the tibia
   IIc: fractures of distal femur and tibial plateau [13]
3. *Bohn-Durbin classification*:
   Type I: double-shaft pattern of fracture
   Type II: the juxta-articular pattern of fracture
   Type III: the epiphyseal pattern of fracture [14]
4. *Letts and Vincent classification*:
   Closed fracture:
   Type A: diaphyseal fractures of both bones
   Type B: metaphyseal fracture of one bone and diaphyseal fracture of the other
   Type C: epiphyseal fracture of one bone and diaphyseal fracture of the other
   Open fracture:
   Type D: only one fracture open
   Type E: both fractures open [9]

8.6   Indications

8.6.1   Conservative or Operative?

Early reports favored nonoperative treatment. However, functional results were not satisfactory in most of the patients, such as nonunion or malunion [15]. The reasons for the conservative therapy included no available internal fixation techniques to provide the desired stability; the incidence of open injuries was high and the disastrous results of internal fixation raised concerns; and considering the complex multisystem injury, the surgeon preferred life over limb. With improved resuscitation techniques and internal fixation devices, more aggressive early stabilization of both fractures is recommended. Surgical stabilization of both fractures produces the best clinical outcomes [16]. Early stabilization is important to prevent systemic complications in polytrauma patients and is facilitated for movement and care [17].

The surgical method should be individualized for each patient. A comprehensive assessment of the fracture type, soft tissue condition, surgical devices available, the surgeon's preference, and the patient's general condition is necessary in order to make individualized treatment strategies.

8.6.2 Time to Intervention

Early studies showed that definitive fixation within 24 h had a positive outcome [18]. However, the associated life-threatening injuries to the head, chest, and abdomen should be managed first in emergency. Meanwhile soft tissue conditions and neurovascular injury may not be ignored. Immediate definitive stabilization of both fractures is possible but may not be indicated for all patients. The hemodynamically stable patients may be indicated for definitive fixation. Polytrauma patients are unable to undergo additional surgical injuries, and damage control orthopedics (DCO) should be the treatment of choice [19, 20]. Temporary external fixation is a suitable alternative to stabilize the entire limb. Internal fixation can be carried out within a week considering the general condition and soft tissue status.

The absolute indications for immediate orthopedic intervention are open fractures, associated with vascular injury or compartment syndrome.

8.6.3 The Choice for Children

The treatment of floating knee in children is controversial. Most authors suggest operative treatment of at least the femoral fracture in patients older than 10 years of age [21]. Conservative methods with closed reduction and casting or splinting are carried out only for younger children. Letts recommended that even in younger patients (less than 9 years old) at least one fracture must be rigidly fixed [9]. Recent

studies reported that both fractures should be treated operatively in all age groups [22].

8.6.4 Treatment of Ligament Injuries

Knee ligaments injury is common. However, early diagnosis is difficult and the assessment is possible only after skeletal stabilization. For pure incomplete collateral ligament injury, conservative treatment is preferred. Avulsion fractures of cruciate ligaments either from femur or tibia should be repaired at an early stage, while the anterior or posterior cruciate ligament (ACL or PCL) reconstruction can be delayed after union of the fractures [5, 6].

8.7 Surgical Technique(s) (Anesthesia, Patient Positioning, Surgical Approach(es), Reduction and Fixation Technique(s))

8.7.1 Adults

Floating knee entails multiple operative sites and usually requires along surgical time. General anesthesia is usually recommended because it is safer and allows for control of the patient's general condition. A sterile tourniquet can be applied in some situations when dealing with tibia fracture, but in most patients it is contraindicated since the femur is also involved.

Patient positioning depends on the surgical plan. Supine position with a pad under the knee on a radiolucent table is the most common setup. It is suitable for femoral and tibial plating, retrograde femoral nailing, tibial nailing, and external fixation. However, when antegrade femoral nailing is indicated, traction position is required (Fig. 8.3). To avoid traction force affecting the definite fixation in tibia, we suggest nailing the femur first with traction and temporary external fixation of the tibia.

Fig. 8.3 Traction
position for femoral
antegrade
intramedullary nail
with external fixation in
tibia

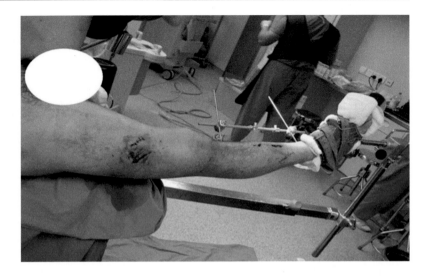

Reduction is one of the most challenging steps of the surgery. The goals of reduction of floating knee are restoration of the alignment of lower limb and anatomic reduction of the articular fragments. To achieve realignment of femur and tibia, we recommend various closed reduction techniques, including traction, clamp, half pin, bone hook, etc. To achieve anatomic reduction of the articular fracture, open reduction under direct vision remains the standard method. In terms of reduction sequence, there is no definite guideline. We suggest starting from the simple fracture site with preserved landmarks.

The decision of reduction strategy and fixation pattern should be made cautiously according to the characteristic of each individual case. For typical "true" floating knee, retrograde femoral nail plus tibial nail is usually a good indication, with fixation of both bones through a single knee incision. This will reduce the surgical time (Fig. 8.4). Ostrum reported 88 % good or excellent results with a full range of knee motion using the above technique [23]. The femoral shaft fracture is addressed first. Stabilization of the femur allows for mobilization of the patient without traction and adequate flexion of the knee, in order to approach the proximal tibial entry point. However, if the femoral fracture extends to the proximal third of the shaft, antegrade nailing is recommended for the femur

(Fig. 8.5). With simultaneous external fixation in the tibia, the surgical technique of antegrade nailing is comparable to isolated femoral fracture. The total surgical time for both femoral and tibial fixation should be under 3 h; if one or both fractures are too complex, a staged strategy is reasonable. Locking plates provide strong stability for metaphyseal fractures and can achieve anatomic reduction with or without free compression lag screws. When the fracture involves the metaphyseal or articular part, locking plates and screws can be applied in this side combined with intramedullary nailing in the diaphyseal side (Fig. 8.6). A minimally invasive approach for the locking plates is strongly recommended in order to preserve the blood supply. In 21 patients with floating knee injury, Hung et al. treated 16 cases of type II or "variant" injury with plates and screws [24]. The authors concluded that when the knee joint is involved, intramedullary nailing is not recommended. Plate fixation can offer anatomic reduction of the articular surface, allowing for early mobilization and maximizing the functional outcome. Different fixation techniques can be combined according to the personality of the fracture. Commonly intramedullary nailing is combined with additional plating for segmental fractures involving the metaphysis of the tibia or femur (Fig. 8.5).

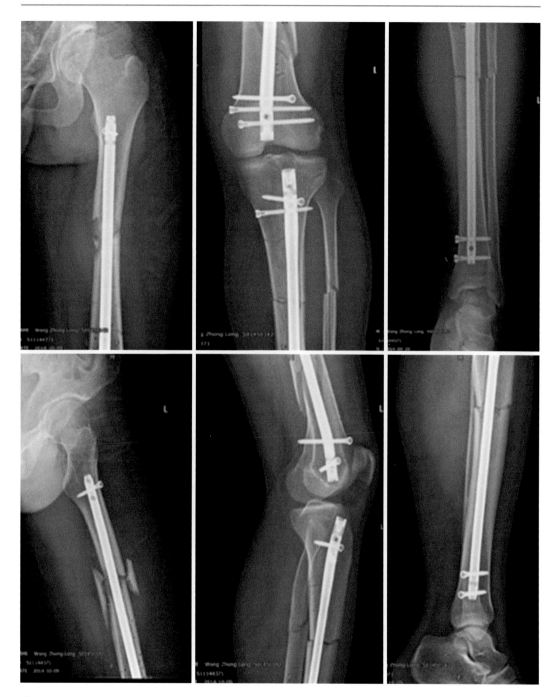

Fig. 8.4 Retrograde nailing for femoral fracture and nailing for tibial fracture

8.7.2 Children

An increasing number of authors noticed the different results of children treated by conservative or surgical methods. They suggested rigid stabilization for both femoral and tibia fracture in older children (>9 years old) and at least one bone fixation in younger patients (<9 years old)

Fig. 8.5 The femoral fracture site extended to upper one third of shaft. Antegrade nailing for femur and nail with additional reduction plate for tibial segmental fracture

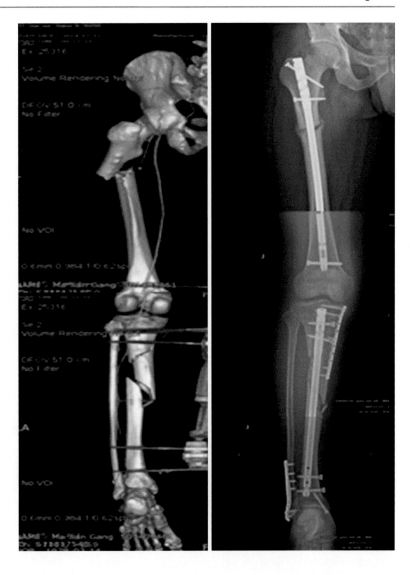

[14, 25, 26]. The surgical technique is generally similar to adults but with attention to preserve the growth plates. Operative treatment options include flexible nails, plates, or external fixators for diaphyseal fractures and crossed K-wires in epiphyseal or metaphyseal fractures. Individual fracture features should always be taken into consideration, and in some cases different fixation techniques can be combined. For example, for an overweight child with closed transverse femoral shaft fracture and proximal tibial fracture, we chose compressive plating for femoral fracture and lateral plate combined with external fixator for the tibia medially to share the stress (Fig. 8.7).

8.8 Postoperative Regimen

Thromboprophylaxis should be started in all patients during the postoperative period. Physiotherapy including early range of motion (ROM) exercises or continuous passive motion is started within 1 week after surgery. Isometric exercises for quadriceps and isotonic for hamstring are allowed as tolerated. For 6 weeks after surgery, weight bearing is not allowed. Then weight bearing is progressively increased as femoral and tibial calluses become evident. Full weight bearing is allowed only after solid continuous callus is evident on routine follow-up radiographs.

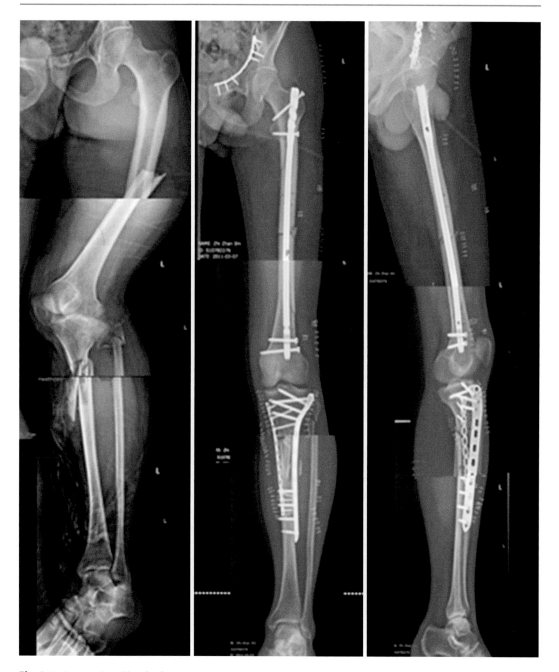

Fig. 8.6 Antegrade nailing for femoral segmental fracture and locking plates for tibial metaphyseal fracture

8.9 Complications

8.9.1 Pulmonary Embolism

Intramedullary nailing is a widely used method for treating the floating knee but has a systemic physiological effects known as "second-hit phenomena." This phenomenon results in increased chances of pulmonary complications especially in polytrauma patients [27, 28]. Canal reaming and insertion of the nail liberate medullary fat with the risk of pulmonary embolism, which can be

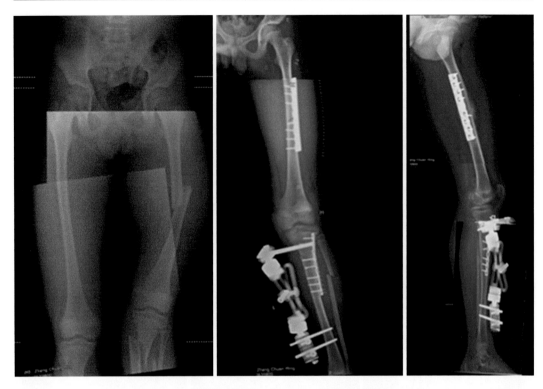

Fig. 8.7 An overweight 15-year-old child with mixed fixation technique. Compressive plate for femoral shaft fracture and lateral locking plate combined with external fixation for proximal tibial fracture

life-threatening because of a fragile respiratory state secondary to the initial trauma.

Cerebral injury has been found to be associated with high risk of pulmonary complications. Poole et al. [29] in a comparison study on lower extremity fracture fixation in head-injured patient found that surgical stabilization of fractures within 24 h of injury reduced the risk of pulmonary complications (fat embolism, pneumonia, and adult respiratory distress syndrome).

8.9.2 Delayed Union or Nonunion

This complication always results from infection or hardware failure. Patients with delayed union/nonunion need either dynamization of the nail or removal of the external fixator and functional bracing of the fracture.

8.9.3 Amputations

This is probably related to the severity of trauma, massive soft tissue crushing, and delay in presentation at the emergency room.

8.9.4 Malunion

Malunion can occur in open fractures and comminuted fractures treated by external fixation. In order to reduce the number of malunions, comminution must be addressed accurately by the use of lag screws. Ipsilateral nailing of femoral and tibial shafts increases the risk of malunion, rotatory instability due to shortening, and axial malalignment. Braten et al. [30] and Sojbjerg et al. [31] found this complication in 21 of 110 patients and 8 of 40 patients, respectively. In order to reduce malunion, preliminary alignment by reduction and manipulation of tibial and femoral fractures facilitates reaming and avoids damage to the medullary canal.

8.9.5 Ankylosis

Intra-articular injury or delayed range of motion of the knee joint may lead to ankylosis. Bonnevialle et al. reported a 15 % rate of knee ankylosis in cases of ipsilateral femoral and tibial fractures. Recently, Hwan Tak et al. [16] reported a 29 % rate of knee ankylosis out of 89 patients. These patients always needed a second soft tissue release surgery.

8.9.6 Instability of the Knee

We suggest to check for meniscal and ligament injuries at the end of the surgery and, when present, plan an early treatment. Vangsness et al. encountered many cases of meniscal and ligament injuries, with a rate of 25 % of meniscal lesions and 50 % of knee instability.

8.10 Results

Some authors reported good results after internal fixation of both fracture sites. This technique has been followed by many orthopedic surgeons. The technique reduced length problems, angular malunion, and secondary interventions following conservative treatment for floating knees in childhood. However, although internal fixation is an excellent treatment, complications and mortality are still high.

The associated injuries and the type of fracture (open, intra-articular, comminution) are prognostic indicators in the floating knee.

Earlier return to activities and excellent/good long-term functional results were observed among patients treated with intramedullary nailing. External fixation of the fractured femur can result in decreased range of movement at the knee due to quadriceps muscle fixation.

The patient with vascular injury has a delay in rehabilitation and a poor final outcome. Vascular injuries associated with the floating knee are a poor prognostic indicator and should be assessed and managed with care [32].

Knee ligament injuries are easily missed due to the "distracting" nature of a floating knee injury. Appropriate management of the knee ligament injury is essential for a good outcome after treatment of the floating knee. Szalay et al. in their study of 34 floating knees found detectable ligament laxity in 53 % of the cases [5]. The Lachmann test is almost 100 % diagnostic of anterior cruciate ligament tear when performed under anesthesia. Moore et al. [33] found that when knee ligament injuries were repaired, a better range of motion was achieved in femoral fractures. They recommended surgical stabilization of the fracture, stress testing of knee ligaments, acute arthroscopy, and ligament repair. Karlström and Olerud criteria are the most widely used in assessing the function of the floating knee (Table 8.1).

Table 8.1 Karlström and Olerud criteria for functional assessment after management of floating knee

Criterion	Excellent	Good	Acceptable	Poor
Symptoms from the thigh or leg	None	Intermittent slight symptoms	More severe symptom impairing function	Considerable functional impairment pain at rest Same as above
Symptoms from knee or ankle joint	None	Same as above	Same as above	Same as above
Walking and sports	Unimpaired	Same as above	Walking distance restricted	Use cane, crutch, or other support
Work and sports	Same as above	Given up sport; work same as before	Change to less strenuous work	Permanent disability
Angulation, rotational deformity, or both	0	<10°	10–20°	>20°
Shortening	0	<1 cm	1–3 cm	>3 cm
Restricted joint mobility	0	<10° at the ankle; <20° at the hip, knee, or both	10–20° at the ankle; 20–40° at the hip, knee, or both	>20° at the ankle; >20° at the hip, knee, or both

References

1. Blake R, McBryde A Jr (1975) The floating knee: ipsilateral fractures of the tibia and femur. South Med J 68:13–16
2. Dwyer AJ, Paul R, Mam MK et al (2005) Floating knee injuries: long-term results of four treatment methods. Int Orthop 29:314–318
3. Paul GR, Sawka MW, Whitelaw GP (1990) Fractures of the ipsilateral femur and tibia: emphasis on intra-articular and soft tissue injury. J Orthop Trauma 4:309–314
4. Adamson GJ, Wiss DA, Lowery GL et al (1992) Type II floating knee: ipsilateral femoral and tibial fractures with intraarticular extension into the knee joint. J Orthop Trauma 6:333–339
5. Szalay MJ, Hosking OR, Annear P (1990) Injury of knee ligament associated with ipsilateral femoral shaft fractures and with ipsilateral femoral and tibial shaft fractures. Injury 21:398–400
6. van Raay JJ, Raaymakers EL, Dupree HW (1991) Knee ligament injuries combined with ipsilateral tibial and femoral diaphyseal fractures: the "floating knee". Arch Orthop Trauma Surg Archiv fur orthopadische und Unfall-Chirurgie 110:75–77
7. Rethnam U, Yesupalan RS, Nair R (2009) Impact of associated injuries in the floating knee: a retrospective study. BMC Musculoskelet Disord 10:7
8. Rios JA, Ho-Fung V, Ramirez N et al (2004) Floating knee injuries treated with single-incision technique versus traditional antegrade femur fixation: a comparative study. Am J Orthop 33:468–472
9. Letts M, Vincent N, Gouw G (1986) The "floating knee" in children. J Bone Joint Surg 68:442–446
10. Davenport HT (1988) Preparations for anaesthesia for the aged. In: Davenport HT, editor. Anaesthesia in the aged patient. Blackwell Scientific publications pp. 183–203
11. Vowles KDJ (1988) Surgical decision in the aged. In: Davenport HT, editor. Anaesthesia in the aged patient. Blackwell Scientific publications pp. 168–182.
12. McHenry TP, Holcomb JB, Aoki N et al (2002) Fractures with major vascular injuries from gunshot wounds: implications of surgical sequence. J Trauma 53:717–721
13. Fraser RD, Hunter GA, Waddell JP (1978) Ipsilateral fracture of the femur and tibia. J Bone Joint Surg 60-B:510–515
14. Bohn WW, Durbin RA (1991) Ipsilateral fractures of the femur and tibia in children and adolescents. J Bone Joint Surg Am 73(3):429–439
15. Karlström G, Olerud S (1977) Ipsilateral fracture of the femur and tibia. J Bone Joint Surg Am 59:240–243
16. Hee HT, Wong HP, Low YP et al (2001) Predictors of outcome of floating knee injuries in adults: 89 patients followed for 2–12 years. Acta Orthop Scand 72:385–394
17. Hung SH, Chen TB, Cheng YM et al (2000) Concomitant fractures of the ipsilateral femur and tibia with intra-articular extension into the knee joint. J Trauma 48:547–551
18. Bone LB, Johnson KD, Weigelt J et al (1989) Early versus delayed stabilization of femoral fractures. A prospective randomized study. J Bone Joint Surg Am 71:336–340
19. Scalea TM, Boswell SA, Scott JD et al (2000) External fixation as a bridge to intramedullary nailing for patients with multiple injuries and with femur fractures: damage control orthopedics. J Trauma 48:613–621; discussion 621–623

20. Pape HC, Hildebrand F, Pertschy S et al (2002) Changes in the management of femoral shaft fractures in polytrauma patients: from early total care to damage control orthopedic surgery. J Trauma 53:452–461; discussion 461–462

21. Yue JJ, Churchill RS, Cooperman DR, et al (2000) The floating knee in the pediatric patient. Nonoperative versus operative stabilization. Clini Orthop Relat Res 376:124–136

22. Arslan H, Kapukaya A, Kesemenli C et al (2003) Floating knee in children. J Pediatr Orthop 23:458–463

23. Ostrum RF (2000) Treatment of floating knee injuries through a single percutaneous approach. Clin Orthop Relat Res 375:43–50

24. Hung SH, Lu YM, Huang HT et al (2007) Surgical treatment of type II floating knee: comparisons of the results of type IIA and type IIB floating knee. Knee Surg Sports Traumatol Arthrosc 15(5):578–586

25. Yue JJ, Churchill RS, Cooperman DR, Yasko AW, Wilber JH, Thompson GH (2000) The floating knee in the pediatric patient. Nonoperative versus operative stabilization. Clin Orthop Relat Res 376:124–136

26. Beaty JH (2005) Operative treatment of femoral shaft fractures in children and adolescents. Clin Orthop Relat Res 434:114–122

27. Giannoudis PV, Smith RM, Bellamy MC et al (1999) Stimulation of the inflammatory system by reamed and unreamed nailing of femoral fractures. An analysis of the second hit. J Bone Joint Surg 81:356–361

28. Ribet ME (1994) 'Damage control' in trauma surgery. Br J Surg 81:627

29. Poole GV, Miller JD, Agnew SG et al (1992) Lower extremity fracture fixation in head-injured patients. J Trauma 32:654–659

30. Braten M, Terjesen T, Rossvoll I (1993) Torsional deformity after intramedullary nailing of femoral shaft fractures. Measurement of anteversion angles in 110 patients. J Bone Joint Surg 75:799–803

31. Sojbjerg JO, Eiskjaer S, Moller-Larsen F (1990) Locked nailing of comminuted and unstable fractures of the femur. J Bone Joint Surg 72:23–25

32. Rethnam U, Yesupalan RS, Nair R (2007) The floating knee: epidemiology, prognostic indicators & outcome following surgical management. J Trauma Manag Outcomes 1:2

33. Moore TM, Patzakis MJ, Harvey JP Jr (1988) Ipsilateral diaphyseal femur fractures and knee ligament injuries. Clin Orthop Relat Res 232:182–189

Periprosthetic Fractures

9

Gabriele Pisanu, Alessandro Crosio,
and Filippo Castoldi

9.1 Epidemiology

The incidence of periprosthetic knee fractures is increasing and will inevitably rise due to the increased number of total knee arthroplasties (TKA) and patients' life expectancy [1]. The total incidence of periprosthetic knee fractures ranges from 0.3 to 5.5 % for primary TKA and up to 30 % for revision TKA [2–5].

The most common type of periprosthetic fracture around the knee is supracondylar: incidence ranging from 0.3 to 2.5 % after primary surgery, mostly within 2–4 years after surgery, and from 1.6 to 38 % after total knee revision [6–8]. The Mayo Clinic Joint Registry reported an incidence of approximately 2 % (of these 0.9 % occurred during revision surgery and 0.1 % during primary surgery) [9].

Probably the true incidence of intraoperative periprosthetic fractures is underestimated because some of these fractures may go undetected, and maybe those with minimal displacement or those that do not require further intervention are not reported [10].

Periprosthetic tibia fractures are more common than femur fractures [11]. The incidence reported from a Mayo Clinic case series of over 17,000 TKAs is 0.1 % for intraoperative fractures and 0.4 % for postoperative fractures. The incidence is higher after revision surgery [12].

Periprosthetic patella fractures can occur both in resurfaced and in unresurfaced patellae. In unresurfaced patellae fractures are rare with an incidence <0.1 %. The incidence in resurfaced patellae ranges from 0.2 to 21 % [13–15]. The incidence after revision surgery is six times higher than in primary TKA [16]. A case series showed that many of these fractures are asymptomatic (44 %) and mostly occur within 1 or 2 years after surgery [15].

9.2 Clinical Examination

Preoperative examination should be focused on determining the type of TKA, fracture configuration, and bone quality. The patient's general health status is essential to identify risk factors or predisposing conditions and exclude infections or pathological fractures. The traumatic mechanism should be investigated. A careful and comprehensive history should be collected also regarding the function of the TKA before the fracture. A painful knee before the fracture should raise the suspicion of a loose, malpositioned, or infected implant. Inflammatory markers including ESR,

G. Pisanu, MD (✉) • A. Crosio, MD
F. Castoldi, MD
Department of Orthopaedics, CTO Turin Hospital,
University of Torino, Torino, Italy
e-mail: gabriele.pisanu@libero.it;
alessandro.crosio@gmail.com;
filippo.castoldi@unito.it

© Springer International Publishing Switzerland 2016
F. Castoldi, D.E. Bonasia (eds.), *Fractures Around the Knee*, Fracture Management Joint by Joint,
DOI 10.1007/978-3-319-28806-2_9

CRP, and white blood cell count should be routinely checked [17].

An accurate physical examination starts from the inspection of the knee that is usually swollen and painful. Palpation of the bone and soft tissue around the TKA can help identify the location of the fracture/s. Neurovascular evaluation as well as stability maneuvers should be carried out.

9.3   Imaging and Preoperative Work-Up

For a correct assessment of the fracture and type and degree of displacement, preoperative imaging should include anteroposterior and lateral x-rays of the femur, tibia, and knee. A comparison with previous x-rays is mandatory and can show pre-existing loosening or malpositioning. Computerized tomography scan is necessary for

defining the comminution of the fracture and the remaining bone stock (Fig. 9.1). Preoperative planning is important to establish the type and size of the primary TKA and if this was stable or not. The choice of implant may be led by the bone stock available for distal fixation.

9.4   Classification

The fractures around TKA can be divided into femoral, tibial, and patellar. These can be intra-operative or postoperative fractures.

Several classifications for periprosthetic femoral fractures have been described: these are based either on the fracture line extension or on the stability of the implant [8, 18–20]. The classification system proposed by Rorabeck et al. is one of the most widely used (Fig. 9.2). The Rorabeck classification system for supracondylar

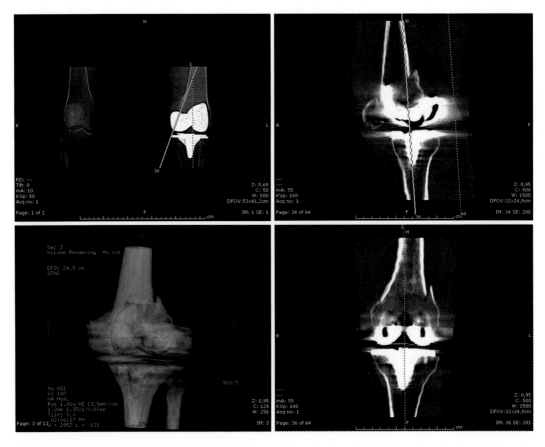

Fig. 9.1 A preoperative CT scan with 3D reconstruction

femoral fractures takes into consideration the fracture displacement and the implant fixation status. It defined three types of fractures: type I, undisplaced fractures around a well-fixed femoral prosthetic component; type II, fractures with a displacement >5 mm or >5° of angulation and a stable femoral prosthetic component (subtype IIB if the fracture is comminuted); and type III, fractures with component loosening or instability and with or without fracture displacement [8]. Su et al. suggested a classification system based on the height of the fracture line relative to the femoral component [19]. Kim has also proposed a new classification which takes into account volume and density of the bone in the distal fracture fragment, reducibility of the fracture, fixation status, and position of the components [20].

Periprosthetic tibia fractures can be classified into four types and three subtypes, according to Felix classification (Fig. 9.3). This widely used classification is based on the fixation status of tibial component and site of the fracture. Type I fractures occur at the tibial plateau, type II are adjacent to the tibial stem, type III occur distal to the prosthetic stem, and type IV involve the tibial tuberosity (subtype A, stable component on x-rays; subtype B, loosening component on x-rays; subtype C, intraoperative fracture) [12].

Three main classification systems have been suggested for periprosthetic patellar fractures, and they are all based on the integrity of the extensor mechanism and stability of the patellar component [14, 15, 21].

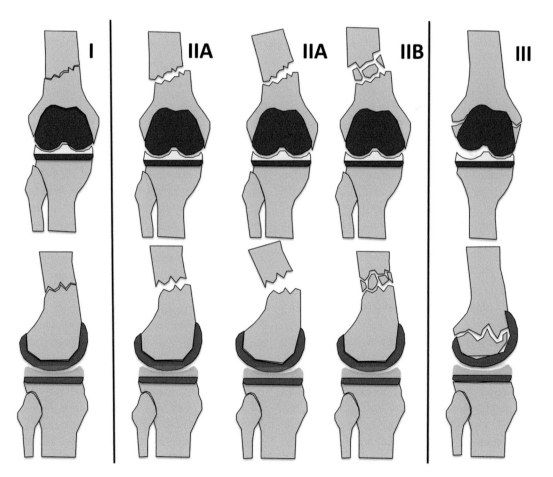

Fig. 9.2 Rorabeck classification: *type I* undisplaced fractures with stable implant, *type IIA* displacement over 5 mm or 5° but stable implant, *type IIB* displaced comminuted fractures, and *type III* displaced or undisplaced fractures with unstable implant

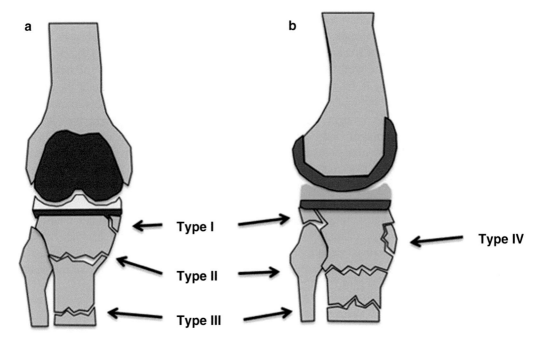

Fig. 9.3 Felix classification: as described in the text, the four types could be divided into (**a**, **b**) according to the stability of the implant at the x-ray examination

Goldberg classified these fractures into the following types: in type I, fractures are located at the periphery of the patella and do not involve the prosthetic component; in type II, the disruption of the extensor mechanism is identified; in type III, the inferior pole is involved (IIIA with ligament rupture, IIIB without ligament rupture); and in type IV, the fracture of the patella is associated with patellofemoral dislocation [14].

9.5   Mechanism and Risk Factors

Intraoperative fractures can be diagnosed and treated immediately. Intraoperative fractures are related frequently to mistakes in surgical technique. Sometimes intraoperative fractures are misdiagnosed and can lead to stress fractures or low-energy bone collapse. Postoperative fractures can occur after low-energy trauma if poor bone quality is present, or after high-energy trauma, especially for tibial fractures.

9.5.1   Femur

Postoperative periprosthetic femur fractures occur mainly after low-energy trauma caused by torsion or compression forces and only sometimes after high-energy trauma [22]. These fractures usually involve the distal third (15 cm) of the femur [2]. In patients with a stemmed femoral component, the forces are transmitted to the tip of the stem, or more proximal region, resulting in more proximal fractures. These fractures may also be the result of an excessive anterior femur resection during surgery. Several studies have demonstrated that anterior femoral notching is associated with femoral supracondylar fractures, occurring in 10–46 % of femurs with notching [2] (Fig. 9.4)

Culp et al. reported that a 3-mm anterior cortical notch resulted in a 30 % reduction in bone strength to torsion, predisposing to the risk of periprosthetic fracture [23]. If anterior femoral notching occurs intraoperatively, sometimes a stemmed femoral component should be implanted to reduce the stress on the anterior femoral cortex,

Fig. 9.4 An example of anterior femoral notch

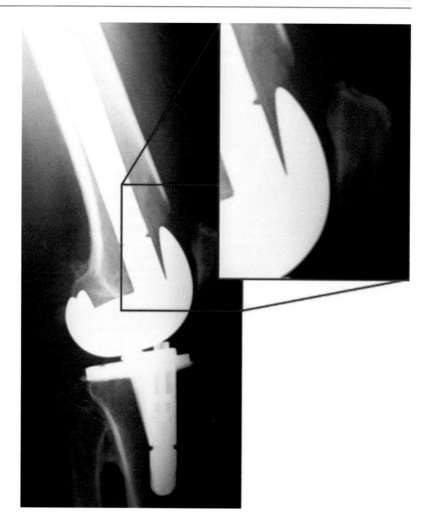

and postoperative weight-bearing should be restricted with the use of walking aids (walker or crutches) if the anterior cortex is markedly compromised.

Intraoperative femoral fractures usually occur when the intramedullary femoral guide is incorrectly positioned (due to the anteriorly bowed shape of the femur). The tip of the guide could penetrate the anterior or anterolateral side of the femoral cortex, generating a fracture. The majority of these fractures may go undetected intraoperatively due to an abundance of soft tissue around the femoral shaft and are only noticed and documented postoperatively from radiographs [24]. For this reason it is very important to plan preoperatively the correct insertion point of the femoral guide, based on the morphology of the femur on anteroposterior and lateral views (Fig. 9.5).

In addition, intercondylar splits or complete fractures of one or both condyles can occur during surgery. These fractures occur quite often in patients with previously diagnosed osteopenia. Technical problems encountered intraoperatively such as improper bone cuts, aggressive impaction of the boxed posterior-stabilized femoral component, and incorrect insertion of the trial component (particularly during revision surgery) can result in fractures [25].

Other risk factors include metal plates or screws previously implanted to fix a fracture or an osteotomy. In two-staged surgeries, hardware must be removed at least 3 months prior to TKA. When hardware removal and TKA are

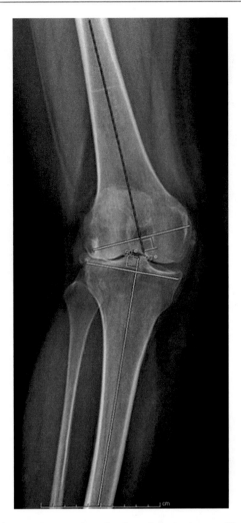

Fig. 9.5 Preoperative planning of the bone cuts. Note that the entry point of the intramedullary guide (*red line*) is not always at the deeper point of the intercondylar notch. It is important to respect preoperative planning in order to avoid fractures of the femoral cortex

performed concurrently, it is preferable to use a long-stemmed prosthesis in order to avoid fractures [26] (Fig. 9.6).

9.5.2 Tibia

Periprosthetic knee fractures of the tibia are more common during revision surgery than during primary surgery. Forceful retraction of a well-fixed tibial component, incorrect cement removal, aggressive impaction of the tibial

component, and osteotomy of the tibial tubercle can result in this type of fracture [12]. In addition, it is important to carefully place the tibial component respecting the axis of the shaft, in order to avoid tibial cortex injury. An eccentric preparation of the tibial canal or malpositioning of the tibial stem can damage the tibial cortex. These fractures are typically vertical and undisplaced.

Postoperative tibial fractures result from acute trauma or fatigue (stress fractures) [11]. These fractures are now quite rare due to the use of keeled or short stem tibial components [27]. Theoretically, the keeled stem with the presence of an intact fibula allows the tibia to withstand substantial torque and shear forces, conveying a mechanical advantage to the bone for the prevention of these fractures as compared to femoral fractures.

9.5.3 Patella

Periprosthetic fractures of the patella can occur due to direct trauma or fatigue. The identified risk factors include rheumatoid arthritis, prolonged steroid use, patellar necrosis, malalignment of the lower limb, malpositioned TKA, and posterior-stabilized implants [28].

These fractures are more frequent in males, because of higher activity levels and weight compared to women [29].

The type of treatment received by the patella during TKA is also a very important factor influencing the outcome (Fig. 9.7). During primary surgery the assistant should manage the patella carefully because excessive stress can cause a patellar fracture or a rupture of the patellar tendon; it is also important, in tight knees, to perform distal femoral resection before patellar lateralization [26].

Heat necrosis and devascularization of the patella during lateral release and excessive Hoffa's fat pad excision could result in damage to the lateral superior genicular artery, increasing the incidence of periprosthetic patella fractures [30]. In addition, asymmetric resection of the patella increases mechanical strain on the joint

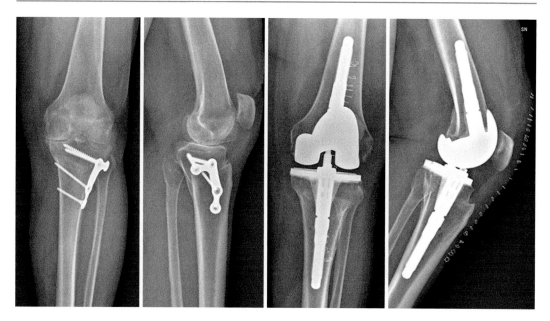

Fig. 9.6 TKA and hardware removal performed concurrently

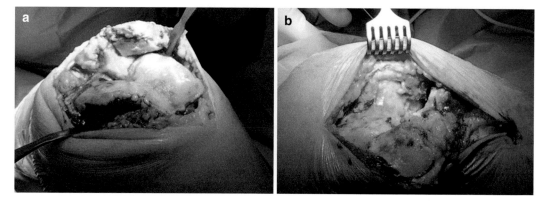

Fig. 9.7 Patella lateralization (**a**) or eversion (**b**)

surface especially when the subchondral bone or the lateral articular surface is included in the resection.

9.6 Treatment and Results

The most appropriate management of periprosthetic knee fractures depends on the patient's general physical condition and pre-fracture ambulatory status; the fracture pattern, location, and displacement; the quality of the bone stock; the presence of other hardware in the proximal femur; the stability of the prosthetic component; and the type of implant [19].

The aim of the treatment is to promote fracture healing within 6 months, recovery of knee range of motion to preinjury level, joint stability, and pain-free function. The surgeon should achieve a minimum range of motion of 90°, less than 5 mm translation, varus/valgus malalignment ≤5°, flexion/extension malalignment ≤10°, minimal rotation, less than 1 cm of femoral shortening, and proper tibiofemoral prosthetic joint alignment [18, 19].

Historically, most periprosthetic fractures were treated conservatively using skeletal traction, casting, or cast bracing. Nonsurgical treatment eliminates surgical risks such as bleeding, infection, loss of fixation, and complications related to anesthesia. A prolonged skeletal traction is not well tolerated and may cause the risks of prolonged recumbency, such as pressure ulcers, atelectasis, pneumonia, pulmonary embolism, deep venous thrombosis, and diffuse muscle atrophy. Long-term immobilization may also result in a loss of knee motion as well as malunion or nonunion [5, 6, 28, 31]. Long-lasting traction treatment is currently obsolete, and the only indications are patients with poor general health status and high operative risks [18, 32]. Although good results were obtained with surgery for periprosthetic knee fracture, a significant incidence of malunion and mechanical failure were described [6]. This is probably due to the vascular damage caused by conventional open plating [33] and the inability to obtain secure fixation in osteoporotic bone. Modern treatment methods addressed these problems. From a surgical standpoint, the technique should be minimally invasive, with the use of implants respecting the vascularity and biology of the healing process, adapting to different TKA designs, and achieving stable fixation in order to allow early motion [34].

9.6.1 Intraoperative Fractures

9.6.1.1 Femur

Fractures of the diaphysis should be treated with a long-stemmed prosthesis with or without bone graft [10]. The stem should bypass the fracture by at least two-to-three femoral canal diameters.

Fractures localized in metaphyseal region are usually vertically oriented, frequently undisplaced, and have intact periosteum [25]. Different authors suggest treating these fractures nonoperatively, with protected weight-bearing and without additional intervention [24].

Displaced intercondylar fractures are infrequent but definitely more complex and difficult to treat. These should be treated with internal fixation by the addition of an intramedullary (IM) stem to the femoral component and trans-

condylar screw fixation. In some cases, the use of single screw fixation was described for these fractures with good results. The single screw is usually sufficient because the cement and femoral prosthesis provide additional stability. We suggest using at least two screws in order to obtain anti-rotational neutralization and to complete the diagnosis with a postoperative CT scan to evaluate the real extension of the fracture.

9.6.1.2 Tibia

As described above this is not a frequent situation. In most of the cases, these fractures are identified postoperatively, and the treatment is weight-bearing protection. In some cases, cancellous screws could be useful to treat a displaced tibial fracture. In rare cases of fractures behind the tip of the stem, cast immobilization and protected weight-bearing are mandatory to allow the healing process [10] (Fig. 9.8).

9.6.2 Postoperative Fractures

The correct treatment is determined after a complete and accurate evaluation and classification of the fracture. Stability of the implant and fracture configuration are the most important aspects guiding the decision-making.

9.6.2.1 Femur

The treatment is based on the Rorabeck and Taylor classifications.

In case of type I, a closed reduction is followed by 4–6 weeks of cast immobilization, followed by a strict follow-up period to monitor the alignment of the fracture every 2 weeks. It is possible to convert in operative treatment if instability appears during follow-up.

This treatment has a success rate between 80 and 100 %. No differences were detected in patient satisfaction between the operative treatment group and nonoperative treatment group for displaced Rorabeck type I fractures (61 vs. 67 %). In the operative treatment group, a higher complication rate was found [7].

Other authors proposed nonoperative treatment in types II and III, but the risk of malunion

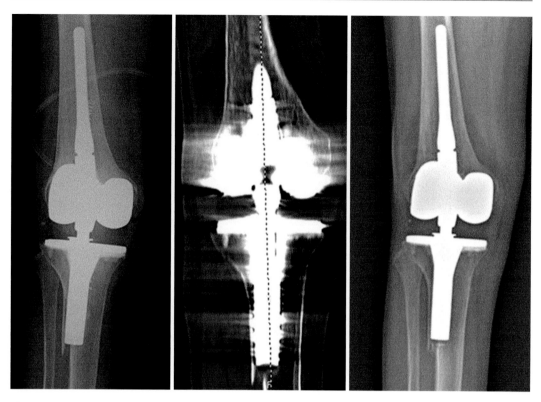

Fig. 9.8 Tibial intraoperative fracture on postoperative x-rays and CT scans. Conservative treatment: x-rays after 5 months

is high [35]. In a study by Moran et al., malunion occurred in all cases after conservative treatment for displaced fractures [36]. Although Chen et al. reported satisfying results in 67 % of cases after conservative treatment in type II fractures, non-operative treatment should be considered only in selected patients with comorbidities, elderly, and with high intraoperative risks [7].

In case of instability of the implant and severely comminute intercondylar fractures, surgery is advisable. If instability is associated with high fracture comminution, revision is required with augment or allograft. In case of instability with large fragments, revision and fracture fixation is the recommended option. In case of fractures with a stable implant but an unstable fracture, an anatomical reduction and rigid fixation are required, allowing early active and passive motion [35].

The surgical treatment could be achieved with different techniques. Fixation can be achieved with intramedullary nails (anterograde or retrograde) and plates with screws.

Nailing

Interlocking intramedullary nailing using interlocking screws is commonly used. Nailing is principally indicated for Rorabeck type II supracondylar femoral fractures. Different studies reported a good healing rate with this technique also compared with plate and screw fixation [37].

Rigid retrograde femoral nails are indicated for fractures with distal fracture fragments large enough to allow insertion of distal screws [37].

Retrograde intramedullary nails should be long enough to reach the level of the lesser trochanter.

Retrograde intramedullary nails can be inserted only with open box femoral component TKAs. For these reasons, retrograde nails cannot be used in patients with posterior-stabilized design prosthesis (Fig. 9.9).

It is important to correctly determine the entry point of the nail. In case of posterior cruciate-retaining knee, the entry point is more posterior than normal because of the femoral component. This can lead to an extension deformity of the knee.

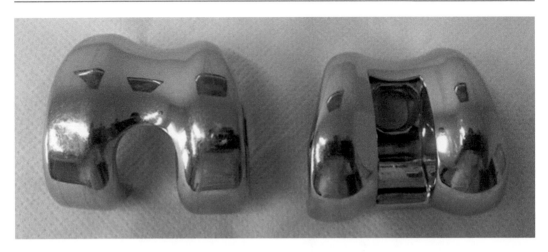

Fig. 9.9 Femoral prosthetic component: cruciate-retaining (*left*) and posterior-stabilized (*right*) designs

The surgical procedure requires an arthrotomy resulting in increased risk of implant infection [37].

Compared to plates, nails have a higher risk of malreduction, including incorrect restoration of length, rotation, and angulation on both coronal and sagittal planes [38].

Advantages of nailing include less soft tissue damage and reduced blood loss compared with conventional metal plate fixation.

Nailing cannot be performed in case of pre-existing intramedullary stem, severe comminution, extremely distal fractures, and unstable TKA. Narrow femoral canals can also be a contraindication for intramedullary nails.

Plate and Screws

Alternative options to treat periprosthetic knee fractures are angled blade plates (ABP), dynamic condylar screws (DCS), and buttress plates [6, 39].

Recently, ORIF with locking periarticular plates became a widely used treatment option, and the introduction of multiple fixed-angle screws allows for optimal fixation around the fracture site and femoral component [40].

Locking plate instrumentation allows for a minimally invasive approach to fracture reduction and implant insertion in order to prevent excessive soft tissue dissection and periosteal stripping. It is possible nowadays to use the new polyaxial designs to vary the insertion angle of the screws (Fig. 9.10).

The patient lies supine with the unaffected leg elevated to allow motion of the C-arm. Usually a lateral approach is required, extended to the distal diaphysis if the fracture extends proximally. The TKA is evaluated and tested for stability. The fracture is then reduced and the plate inserted from distal to proximal using the plate's profile to detach muscles from periosteum. The distal profile is designed to match the lateral condyle. The position is checked with the image intensifier and the first distal screw is inserted. If the reduction is maintained and the plate is in the middle of the shaft the hardware is completed with the other screws. Before closing the capsule, we suggest to copiously irrigate the TKA implant with saline solution (about 2 L). Partial weight-bearing is allowed with crutches for 12 weeks. Early range of motion is allowed.

The outcome is variable and depends on the case series. Some authors reported failure in 30–100 % of cases [5], but with the introduction of locking plates and less invasive stabilization system (LISS), the outcome has greatly improved with rates of complete healing of about 90 % [40].

External Fixation

In periprosthetic knee fractures, the use of the external fixator is infrequent. In an emergency, temporary external fixation could be useful in

Fig. 9.10 Rorabeck II fracture treated with locking plate

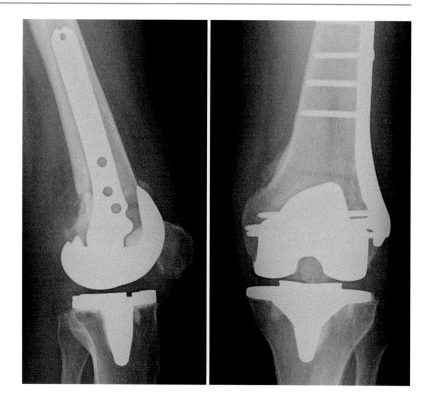

comminuted, exposed, and unstable fractures while awaiting for planning and definitive treatment.

External fixation is not a popular option as a definitive treatment because of problems with quadriceps muscle stripping, limited range of motion of the knee, and risk of infection from pin tracts [23].

Possible indications for the use of hinged external fixator are patients with stable implant and high operative risks [41].

Revision TKA

Revision TKA is necessary in patients with failed implants due to malposition, wear, or loosening (Fig. 9.11). In Rorabeck type II fractures, revision is required when loosening or malpositioning is documented. In Rorabeck type III with poor distal bone stock and implant loosening or malposition, revision is always required.

In elderly patients revision with constrained implants can be considered. In young, active patients, constrained implants are more prone to

loosening. In these cases, the surgeon can restore the bone stock with bone allograft and fracture fixation and then perform the revision in a second step. This option increases the risk of joint stiffness [24].

Another treatment option is the use of an allograft-prosthetic composite (APC). This option could reduce the risk of stiffness but is a complex procedure with higher rate of infection, graft resorption, and component loosening [42].

The reports about revision arthroplasty are good even with fragment fixation. Good outcomes are related to early mobilization and ambulation compared to ORIF [23].

9.6.2.2 Tibia

In fractures involving the tibial plateau, the implant is often loose, and revision TKA is generally recommended with or without metal or bone augmentation of the plateau defect [12].

In fractures around the stem (type II), the implant is usually stable, so nonoperative management is generally sufficient. In loose implants,

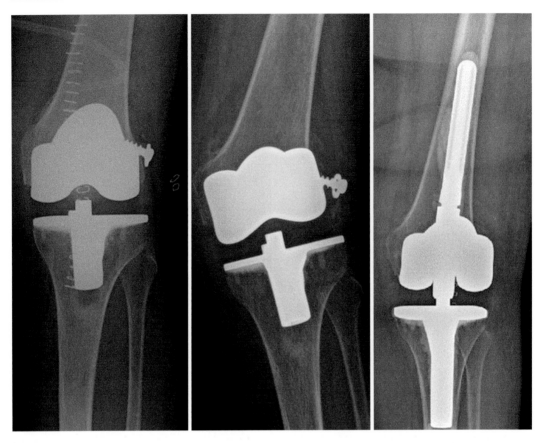

Fig. 9.11 Intraoperative condylar fracture treated with a screw; 1 month after surgery, x-rays showed displacement, and the patient was revised to a constrained implant

revision with long-stemmed tibial components is the treatment of choice. In case of extensive bone loss, allograft is required.

Distal fractures can be managed with reduction and internal fixation if required, but usually the implant is stable.

Particular attention should be paid to subtype IV fractures. These fractures need to be managed carefully because the tibial tuberosity is essential for extensor mechanism function. In these cases, internal fixation with screws is required. In most cases, the tibial component is stable and revision is not required. If revision is required, long-stemmed tibial components are necessary. The stem is inserted before performing fracture reduction and fixation. Many authors also described the use of semitendinosus rerouting to augment the tendon [43].

In revision of the tibial component, the surgeon has to respect different rules: a stemmed tibial component is usually necessary; the stem has to pass the fracture site and give stability to the fracture; the unstable fragments have to be fixed with screws; in proximal tibial fractures, metal augmentations are enough for defects <5 cm; and if bigger defects are present, allograft of tumor prosthesis should be considered [43].

9.6.2.3 Patella

In fractures with stable prosthetic component and extensor mechanism integrity, conservative treatment achieves good results.

Comminuted fractures with prosthetic component stability and/or lesion of the extensor mechanism could be treated with removal of the small fragments and repair of the tendon to the bone with good restoration of the function [15].

In case of instability of the implant, a careful evaluation of residual bone stock is essential. It is possible to perform revision surgery if the bone stock is sufficient; otherwise, hemipatellectomy or total patellectomy is required. Total patellectomy should be reserved to patients with extremely poor bone stock and with highly comminuted fractures.

Nonsurgical treatment should always be considered even in cases with unstable components if the patient has mild symptoms and good knee function. Good results were described with this approach [14].

A systematic review regarding patellar periprosthetic fracture reported a 19 % infection rate and a 92 % rate of nonunion after surgical fixation of patellar fractures with tension band wiring. On the other hand, good results were described in most cases treated not surgically. Range of motion after conservative treatment usually results in 10° of extension lag in and 10–20° of lag in flexion [13].

9.7 Complications

Complications include decreased range of motion, malalignment, infection, and nonunion.

A review of the literature evaluated the complications after periprosthetic femoral fractures. These fractures were managed nonsurgically in 39 % of the cases and surgically in 60 %. In the cases treated conservatively, a higher rate of complications (31 %) was found compared to surgically treated cases (19 %). In the surgical group, complications included infections (3 %), delayed unions or nonunions (7 %), malunions (4 %), hardware failures (3 %), and other complications (3 % intraoperative death, pulmonary embolism, and hardware impingement) [19]. In a metanalysis, complications of patients treated with locking plates included infection (3 %), implant failure (4 %), nonunion (9 %), and revision surgery (13 %). In the conservative group, complications consisted of delayed unions or nonunions (14 %) and malunions (18 %) [34].

In another paper, no difference was found between different nonsurgical management (casting, splinting, bracing, traction) and surgical management (ORIF, intramedullary nailing, external fixation, total knee replacement) [19].

After surgical internal fixation with cerclage wire of periprosthetic patellar fractures, the mean infection rate was 19.2 % and nonunion was 92 % [13].

References

1. Johnston AT, Tsiridis E, Eyres KS, Toms AD (2012) Periprosthetic fractures in the distal femur following total knee replacement: a review and guide to management. Knee 19(3):156–162
2. Healy WL, Siliski JM, Incavo SJ (1993) Operative treatment of distal femoral fractures proximal to total knee replacements. J Bone Joint Surg Am 75:27–34
3. Inglis AE, Walker PS (1991) Revision of failed knee replacements using fixed-axis hinges. J Bone Joint Surg Br 73:757–761
4. Ritter MA, Faris PM, Keating EM (1988) Anterior femoral notching and ipsilateral supracondylar femur fractures in total knee arthroplasty. J Arthroplasty 3:185–187
5. Figgie MP, Goldberg VM, Figgie HE III et al (1990) The results of treatment of supracondylar fracture above total knee arthroplasty. J Arthroplasty 5:267–276
6. Merkel KD, Johnson EW Jr (1986) Supracondylar fracture of the femur after total knee arthroplasty. J Bone Joint Surg Am 68:29–43
7. Chen F, Mont MA, Bachner RS (1994) Management of ipsilateral supracondylar femur fractures following total knee arthroplasty. J Arthroplasty 9:521–526
8. Rorabeck CH, Taylor JW (1999) Periprosthetic fractures of the femur complication total knee arthroplasty. Orthop Clin North Am 30:265–277
9. Berry DJ (1990) Periprosthetic fractures after major joint replacement. Epidemiology: hip and knee. Orthop Clin North Am 30:183–190
10. Engh GA, Ammeen DJ (1997) Periprosthetic fractures adjacent to total knee implants. Treatment and clinical results. J Bone Joint Surg Am 79:1100–1113
11. Rand JA, Coventry MB (1980) Stress fractures after total knee arthroplasty. J Bone Joint Surg Am 62:226–233
12. Felix NA, Stuart MJ, Hanssen AD (1997) Periprosthetic fractures of the tibia associated total knee arthroplasty. Clin Orthop 345:113–124
13. Chalidis BE, Tsiridis E, Tragas AA et al (2007) Management of periprosthetic patellar fractures: a systematic review of the literature. Injury 38:714–724
14. Goldberg VM, Figgie HE 3rd, Inglis AE, Figgie MP, Sobel M, Kelly M, Kraay M (1988) Patellar fracture

type and prognosis in condylar total knee arthroplasty. Clin Orthop Relat Res 236:115–122

15. Ortiguera CJ, Berry DJ (2002) Patellar fracture after total knee arthroplasty. J Bone Joint Surg Am 84: 532–540

16. Grace JN, Sim FH (1988) Fracture of the patella after total knee arthroplasty. Clin Orthop Relat Res 230: 168–175

17. Greidanus NV, Masri BA, Garbuz DS, Wilson SD, McAlinden MG, Xu M et al (2007) Use of erythrocyte sedimentation rate and C-reactive protein level to diagnose infection before revision total knee arthroplasty. A prospective evaluation. J Bone Joint Surg Am 89-A:1409–1416

18. Digioia AM 3rd, Rubash HE (1991) Periprosthetic fractures of the femur after total knee arthroplasty. A literature review and treatment algorithm. Clin Orthop Relat Res 271:135–142

19. Su ET, DeWal H, Di Cesare PE (2004) Periprosthetic femoral fractures above total knee replacements. J Am Acad Orthop Surg 12:12–20

20. Kim K, Egol KA, Hozack WJ et al (2006) Periprosthetic fractures after total knee arthroplasties. Clin Orthop Rel Res 446:167–175

21. Parvizi J, Kim KI, Oliashirazi A et al (2006) Periprosthetic patellar fractures. Clin Orthop Relat Res 446:161–166

22. Bezwada HP, Neubauer P, Baker J et al (2004) Periprosthetic supracondylar femur fractures following total knee arthroplasty. J Arthroplasty 19:453–458

23. Culp RW, Schmidt RG, Hanks G, Mak A, Esterhai JL Jr, Heppenstall RB (1990) Supracondylar fracture of the femur following prosthetic knee arthroplasty. Clin Orthop 252:182–189

24. Parvizi J, Jain N, Schmidt A (2008) Periprosthetic knee fractures. J Orthop Trauma 22:663–671

25. Lombardi AV, Mallory TH, Waterman RA et al (1995) Intercondylar distal femoral fracture. An unreported complication of posterior-stabilized total knee arthroplasty. J Arthroplasty 10:643–650

26. Backstein D, Safir O, Gross A (2007) Periprosthetic fractures of the knee. J Arthroplasty 22(4 Suppl 1):45–49

27. Lotke PA, Ecker ML (1977) Influence of positioning of prosthesis in total knee replacement. J Bone Joint Surg Am 59:77–79

28. Cain PR, Rubash HE, Wissinger HA et al (1986) Periprosthetic femoral fractures following total knee arthroplasty. Clin Orthop 208:205–214

29. Zalzal P, Backstein D, Gross AE (2006) Notching of the anterior femoral cortex during total knee arthroplasty characteristics that increase local stresses. J Arthroplasty 21:737–743

30. Le AX, Cameron HU, Otsuka NY, Harrington IJ, Bhargava M (1999) Fracture of the patella following total knee arthroplasty. Orthopedics 22:395–398

31. Sisto DJ, Lachiewicz PF, Insall JN (1985) Treatment of supracondylar fractures following prosthetic arthroplasty of the knee. Clin Orthop 196:265–272

32. Mittlmeier T, Stockle U, Perka C, Schaser KD (2005) Periprosthetic fractures after total knee joint arthroplasty. Unfallchirurg 108:481–495

33. Farouk O, Krettek C, Miclau T, Schandelmaier P, Guy P, Tscherne H (1999) Minimally invasive plate osteosynthesis: does percutaneous plating disrupt femoral blood supply less than traditional technique? J Orthop Trauma 13:401–406

34. Herrera DA, Kregor PJ, Cole PA, Levy BA, Jonsson A, Zlowodzki M (2008) Treatment of acute distal femur fractures above a total knee arthroplasty: systematic review of 415 cases (1981–2006). Acta Orthop 79:22–27

35. Dennis DA (2001) Periprosthetic fractures following total knee arthroplasty. J Bone Joint Surg Am 83: 120–130

36. Moran MC, Brick GW, Sledge CB, Dysart SH, Chien EP (1996) Supracondylar femoral fracture following total knee arthroplasty. Clin Orthop Relat Res 324: 196–209

37. Maniar RN, Umlas ME, Rodriguez JA et al (1996) Supracondylar femoral fracture above a PFC posterior cruciate-substituting total knee arthroplasty treated with supracondylar nailing. A unique technical problem. J Arthroplasty 11:637–639

38. Pao JL, Jiang CC (2005) Retrograde intramedullary nailing for nonunions of supracondylar femur fracture of osteoporotic bones. J Formos Med Assoc 104:54–59

39. Raab GE, Davis CM 3rd (2005) Early healing with locked condylar plating of periprosthetic fractures around the knee. J Arthroplasty 20:984–989

40. Kregor PJ, Hughes JL, Cole PA (2001) Fixation of distal femoral fractures above total knee arthroplasty utilizing the Less Invasive Stabilization System (L.I.S.S.). Injury 32:SC64–SC75

41. Refaat M, Coleman S, Meehan JP, Jamali AA (2015) Periprosthetic supracondylar femur fracture treated with spanning external fixation. Am J Orthop 44(2):90–93

42. Wong P, Gross AE (1999) The use of structural allograft for treating periprosthetic fractures about the hip and knee. Ortho Clin North Am 30:259–264

43. Hanssen AD, Stuart MJ (2000) Treatment of periprosthetic tibial fractures. Clin Orthop Relat Res 380: 91–98

Management of the Complications Following Fractures Around the Knee (Infection and Non-union)

10

Daniele Santoro, Laura Ravera, Corrado Bertolo, Domenico Aloj, and Bruno Battiston

10.1 Femur

In 1957, Watson-Jones noted that 'few injuries present more difficult problems than supracondylar fractures of the femur' [1]. Since then, the development of stabilisation techniques has greatly improved the treatment of these fractures [2–4]. Even after appropriate initial fracture fixation, however, non-union of the distal femur is a potential complication that has been reported in up to 17 % of cases [5–19]. Although relatively uncommon because of the excellent perfusion and the abundant cancellous bone surfaces [20, 21], the failure of a distal femur synthesis remains a difficult problem to deal with.

Distal femoral fractures arise from two main mechanisms of injury [22]. These are caused either by high-energy traumas, such as road traffic accidents, which may lead to open injuries

with considerable comminution of the condyles and metaphysis, or by low-energy traumas, in elderly populations with severe osteoporosis.

The possible presence of total-knee prosthesis represents a major challenge: the periprosthetic fracture is a very difficult task in terms of bone grip, fracture fixation, possibilities of preserving the prosthesis and, therefore, high risk of local complications and fixation failure. No consensus exists on the management of either type of distal femoral fracture [23]. Before the introduction of the concept of stable fixation by the AO, supracondylar fractures of the femur were often treated not surgically by means of skeletal traction [24].

The therapeutic strategy is based on the restoration of limb length, articular surface, rotational alignment and early mobilisation [22, 23, 25, 26].

The management is often complicated by the small size and poor bone quality of the distal fragment and the presence of bone loss with shortening, angulation, rotational deformity and contamination. As the optimal stability is a purpose not so easy to reach, in the past the knee motion was too often restricted to avoid an overstress at the fracture site. If this protected the small fragment fixation, it led to high stresses across the metaphysis. The only solution for the orthopaedic surgeons was to increase the use of internal fixation hardware.

Infection remains a significant issue in high-energy peri-articular fractures of the knee. In

D. Santoro, MD (✉) • B. Battiston, MD
"Città della Salute e della Scienza",
CTO Hospital, Ortopedia e Traumatologia 3,
Via Zuretti 29, Torino 10126, Italy
e-mail: dasantoro@cittadellasalute.to.it

L. Ravera, MD • C. Bertolo, MD
"Città della Salute e della Scienza",
Clinica Universitaria Ortopedia e Traumatologia,
CTO Hospital, Via Zuretti 29, Torino 10126, Italy

D. Aloj, MD
"Città della Salute e della Scienza",
Ortopedia e Traumatologia Universitaria,
CTO Hospital, Via Zuretti 29, Torino 10126, Italy

© Springer International Publishing Switzerland 2016
F. Castoldi, D.E. Bonasia (eds.), *Fractures Around the Knee*, Fracture Management Joint by Joint,
DOI 10.1007/978-3-319-28806-2_10

high-level trauma centres, infection rates after distal femoral fractures are <5 % [27]. In this anatomical region, the bone is notably vulnerable to infection due to a lack of muscle coverage and limited vascular supply. The metallic implants are a favourable environment for bacterial adherence. The possible implication is the need for an aggressive debridement and the removal of fixation devices.

Non-union of distal femoral fractures is uncommon but difficult to treat. The incidence varies from 0 % to 6 % following internal fixation [13, 28–30]. This was about 25 % in the 1970s [12].

Very little data have been published on the management of distal femoral non-unions. Casts and braces used in the past for the management of these cases resulted in increased muscle atrophy and joint stiffness, further decreasing the possibility of bone healing [7, 31]. A 95° fixed angle blade plate or a dynamic condylar screw (DCS) plate with or without bone graft has been frequently used [15, 32, 33].

In the past, some authors suggested that open reduction after debridement of the non-union site followed by internal fixation and bone grafting can lead to successful results, whereas others recommended the addition of cortical strut allograft [33–36]. Wang and Weng [36] retrospectively evaluated 13 patients with distal femoral non-unions treated with internal fixation and strut allograft. The union rate was 100 %, and the post-operative knee motion was 71° on average.

Supracondylar nails have not shown successful outcomes in terms of union rate with frequent nail breakage [37–40].

Trans-articular fixation of the knee joint using a Kuntscher nail has been described, but, although good union rates were achieved, the knee stiffness caused discomfort and severe limitations to the patients [41]. In Beall's [41] study, the ROM was only 49° after the nail was removed and the infection rate was 25 %. The knee joint immobilisation was also proposed by Scuderi [15] who immobilised the joint by means of post-operative traction for up to 3 months.

When compared with such an aggressive strategy, the blade plate resulted in excellent outcomes in terms of union rate and function, but it can be considered inadequate by current standards.

External fixators have shown an optimal approach to soft tissues and offered good results in handling infected and complex non-unions [15, 42–44]. They also allow for a proximal or mid-diaphyseal corticotomy: this can be useful when a large piece of bone has been removed, and this gap needs to be filled by means of distraction osteogenesis. In addition to lengthening, external fixators can be used to correct angulation, translation and rotation [45].

Metaphyseal fractures including distal femoral fractures have a good intrinsic healing capacity because of abundant physiological blood supply [46]. This was described by Charnley and Baker [47]. Problems in metaphyseal region may arise because of gaps due to bone loss or tissue interposition (biomechanical), excessive motion at the fracture site (mechanic), infection or even the presence of synovial fluid coming from the disrupted capsule (biological) [46]. In the distal femur, unique anatomical features (short distal fragment, proximity to the knee joint, poor bone stock and the traction by the gastrocnemius muscle) can contribute to distal femoral nonunion [15].

The complex non-union healing can lead to several operations, worsening the soft-tissue coverage, scarring and causing additional joint stiffness.

The principles of management of distal femoral non-unions should be the same of non-union treatment as described by Zum Brunnen and Brindley in 1968: reduction of fragments, adequate fixation, healing of soft tissues and stimulation of osteogenesis [48]. Saleh in 1992 summarised these principles in the triad realignment, stabilisation and stimulation [49].

Internal fixation causes deep soft-tissue dissection and periosteal stripping, further impairing the blood supply. Antegrade and supracondylar nails minimally disturb the soft-tissue envelope. Sometimes, the nail does not provide adequate stability [37, 40]. External fixation is an optimal solution when biology is the main issue [45].

Wu [37] noted that in the distal non-unions treated with the antegrade nails, only one locking screw can usually be inserted. This is inadequate for rigid fixation because of the short segment, wide canal, thin cortices and often poor bone quality: two out of seven nails broke in their case series. In Koval's study [40], using the supracondylar nail, eight out of 16 nails broke and union was achieved only in 25 % of patients. Chapman [33] advocated the anterior approach for internal fixation in order to preserve the blood supply with exposure of only the anterolateral surface, allow for a better control of the adhesions in the knee region and improve the range of motion.

An early range of motion is crucial to a successful functional outcome.

10.1.1 Plating

ORIF is very effective in restoring alignment and preserving knee motion [6, 9, 10, 13, 14, 28, 50, 51], but can be associated with infection, non-union, implant failure and inadequate correction of the deformity [6, 8, 12, 18, 19, 52].

As distal femur fractures are well addressed by plating techniques [2, 53, 54], non-united fractures should also be approached by a similar technique.

Because of the forces crossing the distal femur, the typical non-union pattern is a varus and/or extension deformity (similar to the acute fracture in this area). The correction of this can be complicated by the small size fragments and the poor bone quality [40, 55, 56].

Several alternative methods have been developed for the treatment of distal femoral non-union because of concerns regarding the high incidence of failure, wound complications and infection after traditional plating procedures [12, 16, 18, 42, 57–60]; among these intramedullary nails [39, 40, 58] minimise soft-tissue dissection and provide a more physiological load-sharing fixation device [21, 37, 40, 61]. However, intramedullary nails can be a suboptimal solution if a deformity needs to be corrected, the distal small fragments require a stable fixation and a dynamic compression across the non-union site is required (this would probably entail a significant shortening) [39, 41, 58]. These issues led to disappointing results, with a high incidence of hardware failure, particularly in low supracondylar non-unions [37, 40, 58]. Furthermore, intramedullary nails often need to be removed [37, 58].

The locking plates were developed by the AO/ASIF in the late 1990s [62, 63]. These systems can be used in the management of complex distal femoral fractures, particularly the AO 33 A1–C3 types [64]. Biomechanical studies suggested that locking plates withstood higher loads, providing a more stable fixation, than condylar buttress plates and dynamic condylar screws latters [65].

Stress tests indicated that the LISS (LISS, Synthes Paoli, PA, USA) provided improved distal fixation of femoral fractures in osteoporotic bone, bearing greater axial loads and requiring higher energy to failure, compared to the angled blade plates or intramedullary nails [66, 67].

The 'fatigue failure' of the osteoporotic implant-bone construct is a serious problem in elderly patients. Standard implants often fail, and this is due to both the weakness of the bone and the critical blood supply. Vascularization can be impaired by the fracture, the surgical approach and the damage to the soft tissues as well as by the compression of the plate over the periosteum. The locking plates address these aspects. The design of these plates with angular stable locking screws acts as an internal fixator, with no need for compression and contact of the plate to the bone surface in order to achieve good stability of the bone-implant construct. This preserves the muscles, soft-tissue envelope and local periosteal blood supply, especially when applied percutaneously. While the classic plate fixation transfers the strain in an axial loading, the locking plates transfer the load to the screws along the bone axis [63, 68, 69]. In addition, the locking screws account for an excellent grip also in the osteoporotic bone [69].

The main concerns about compression plating of distal femoral non-unions are the exposure and the consequent bone devascularization, with an increased risk of non-union and infection [12, 17, 18, 32, 42, 57, 60, 70, 71]. The 'sparing tissue approach' used in acute fractures has been implemented in non-unions too. Indirect reduction techniques [2, 54, 72] have been developed, reducing the need for non-union exposure and focusing on acceptable axial alignment without anatomic reduction of non-articular fragments.

10.1.2 External Fixation

A short distal fragment, poor bone quality and compromised soft tissues are associated with poor outcomes. Healing may be achieved with deformity and leg-length discrepancy leading to post-traumatic osteoarthritis and stiffness of the knee [34, 37, 73, 74]. This may lead to arthrodesis [75, 76] and, sometimes, amputation.

Infected non-unions are a real challenge for the orthopaedic surgeon. Bone loss, poor soft-tissue coverage and extensive scars are the usual implications of the bacterial colonisation, and the anatomical and functional outcomes are often affected by deformity, shortening, osteoarthritis and stiffness.

Ilizarov techniques [70, 77–83] minimise dissection while allowing for gradual (or immediate) correction of deformity, compression across the non-union, stable fixation of the distal fragment and immediate post-operative weight bearing. These advantages are, however, tempered by a significant learning curve, high incidence of complications, need for frequent re-operation, poor patient tolerance and frequent outpatient examinations [70].

The Ilizarov frame tolerates easily torsion and bending, allowing axial compression during physiological walking [80, 81].

In 1951, Ilizarov began to use distraction osteogenesis to treat acute fractures [78–80]. Over the years, knowledge and tools have evolved, and indications have been extended to associated complications: non-union, chronic osteomyelitis, shortening, joint contracture and deformity.

The Ilizarov strategy for infected non-union is based on the removal of infected tissues and bone debridement/resection, stabilisation with ring fixators and restoration of bone defect by means of distraction osteogenesis. When the bone gap is restored, the residual deformity can be corrected and the docking site compressed.

Distraction osteogenesis and bone transport form new, strong and resistant bone. In the presence of infection, the healthy regenerated bone delivers antibiotics locally and increases the possibility of infection eradication [84].

Complex regional pain syndrome and soft-tissue atrophy is minimised by early weight bearing and joint motion [84]. Therefore, the use of Ilizarov technique for infected non-union of the tibia is increasing in popularity [85–87]. Nonetheless, reports describing large series of patients with infected non-union of the femur treated with the Ilizarov technique are rare [88–90].

The results of conventional treatment of infected non-union of the femur are poor, due to the high energy of the trauma, multiple surgeries, late presentation, bone and soft-tissue infection, bone loss, osteoporosis, poor vascularity, associated deformities and shortening. According to Ilizarov, gradual traction on living tissues creates stress that stimulates and maintains regeneration and active growth of tissues (bone, muscle, fascia, tendon, nerve, vessels, skin). This principle is called 'the law of tension stress' [76]. The primary objective of Ilizarov was to treat the infection by means of increased vascularity at the septic site and biological stimulation through the corticotomy ('osteomyelitis burns in the fire of regeneration', he said) [76]. When bone resection and debridement are not performed, the infection is rarely eradicated. Therefore, osteogenesis must be preceded by debridement. New bone sprouts between surfaces are gradually (about 0.5/1 mm per day) pulled apart. Moving bone segments will fill the gap. The trailing end regenerates bone by intramembranous ossification [84]. The damage at the corticotomy site determines the quality and quantity of regeneration: injury to the bone marrow, nutrient artery and its branches and the periosteal soft tissues should be minimised [76]. The quality and quantity of the osteogenesis during distraction depend on the rigidity of bone fragment fixation, the damage at the corticotomy site, the amount of the lengthening and the rhythm of distraction [76]. The biological response of the tissues to distraction is intrinsic, and thus general body anabolism should always be positively maintained [84].

Latency is the time period between corticotomy and the beginning of distraction. Short latency is related to poor regeneration, whereas longer latency facilitates early consolidation and fusion. Depending on the damage during corticotomy, a latency period of 0–14 days is recommended.

During distraction osteogenesis, physiological bone loading and mobilisation are important rules [84]. When the transport is complete, fibrous tissue removal and cancellous bone grafting at the matching bone ends may be required (docking site stimulation) [89, 91, 92] in order to make it heal faster.

The duration of external fixation and any associated complications can be substantially reduced with the technique of multiple segment lengthening and extemporaneous compression at the end of traction [93].

10.1.3 Arthrodesis

A knee arthrodesis may be a preferable alternative in younger patients with recalcitrant distal femoral non-unions; however, this should be reserved for cases where other therapeutic options are not feasible. The most common indication is pain and instability: loss of extensor mechanism, extensive metaphyseal bone loss, ligamentous instability and resistant bacteria are all known indications [94]. Techniques for arthrodesis include intramedullary nailing, plating, external fixation and circular frame constructs. In the presence of extensive bony defects, vascularised fibular grafts, massive allografts, bone cement and distraction osteogenesis should be considered.

Knee fusion provides a more efficient gait in terms of energy consumption, when compared with above-knee amputation, assuming there is a well-functioning foot [95]. The management of large bone defects around the knee is particularly troublesome [96–98].

The cons of intramedullary nails for the treatment of infection are well documented, even when a two-stage approach is performed [99, 100]. Ilizarov technique gives more opportunities in eradicating the infection and optimising the soft-tissue management before definitive treatment. Other advantages over intramedullary or plate fixation include 1) the possibility of early weight bearing, 2) frame modifications to optimise mechanical properties in relation to the healing phase, 3) compression across the arthrodesis site and 4) fine corrections to restore the mechanical and anatomical axis [101]. Complications often arise and patients must be counselled and selected upon their ability to comply. Frames are bulky and pin sites will get often infected requiring antibiotics and occasional pin and wire exchanges. Despite this, the benefit of simultaneous arthrodesis compression, correction of shortening and/or mechanical axis deviation cannot be overlooked. During the initial treatment, weight bearing can be restricted to promote soft-tissue recovery, and therefore the patients are at higher risk of deep vein thrombosis (DVT) [102].

10.2 Tibia

The surgical management of tibial plateau fractures remains a challenge. High-energy tibial plateau fractures are often the result of blunt trauma and associated with soft-tissue problems.

The current surgical options do not guarantee a constant favourable outcome of these injuries. Operative techniques require considerable surgical skills and thorough preoperative evaluation. Schatzker's classification [13] is widely used in guiding the treatment of these fractures. The surgeon must have deep knowledge of the local anatomy, the biomechanics of fracture fixation and patterns of the physiopathology of fracture healing. The surgeon should individualise the operative treatment respecting numerous factors, such as the patient's age, pre-existing levels of activity, medical morbidity and expectations [103]. Injury considerations should include the extent of fracture comminution and joint impaction, associated injuries and condition of the soft tissues. Numerous studies have shown that infection and non-union/malunion are the two most severe complications [13, 103, 104].

Unicondylar and bicondylar plateau fractures in young patients, with good bone stock and a few well-defined articular fragments, do well with modern reduction and internal fixation techniques [104, 105]. Young patients' fractures should be anyway addressed at the best achievable anatomic articular reconstruction, even when the comminution is substantial. This leads the surgeon to opt for a traditional surgical strategy (open submeniscal arthrotomy, the amount of screws and plates depending on the fracture pattern), sometimes associated with an arthroscopic look [106]. When the skin or the soft-tissue conditions do not allow for a traditional ORIF, the metaphyseal fracture can be fixed by means of an external frame, more often circular [106, 107]. The external fixation treatment is commonly accepted only in Schatzker V/VI type fractures, where other indications should be cautiously considered [107].

When the patient is osteopenic, old, with low functional demands, the fracture is bicondylar, largely comminuted, circular external frame, with or without a minimally invasive joint reconstruction, can be a valuable option for the surgeon [106]. In the patients unable to cope with adequate pin care, a functional brace [106], possibly followed by a total-knee arthroplasty, may be preferable [107].

Whether internal or external fixation techniques are used, appropriate management of the soft tissues is the cornerstone in the successful treatment of these injuries. When extensive comminution and compromised soft tissues advise against internal fixation techniques, circular external fixators provide an excellent alternative option, even in young patients.

The goal of internal fixation is to provide stable fixation of a reduced fracture, resistant enough to permit early range of motion. Although the prognosis for surgically treated tibial plateau fractures has improved due to a better understanding of soft-tissue management, preoperative planning and fixation techniques, complications are still common. In a randomised prospective study by Wyrsch et al. [108], 15 operative complications in 7 patients treated with ORIF were described, as opposed to 4 complications in 4 patients managed with external fixation.

The infection rate following ORIF in tibial plateau fractures varies between 2 % [109] and 11 % [110]. A 9 % deep vein thrombosis rate was reported in patients treated nonoperatively, while a 6 % rate in patients treated with ORIF [111].

In a study by Lachiewicz and Funcik [112], 43 displaced tibial plateau fractures were treated by means of ORIF and 14 patients required hardware removal. Fixation failure with wound breakdown and infection is often a disastrous complication that may ultimately lead to a secondary knee arthrodesis.

Hybrid techniques of closed reduction, minimal internal fixation and external fixation have shown lower infection rates compared with internal fixation [113].

It has been observed that, in femur shaft fractures, the risk of contamination is higher if the external fixator screws are maintained for more than 2 weeks. Therefore, converting the bridging fixator to an ORIF before 2 weeks is recommended [114]. As this is not always possible, the screws must be placed far away from the subsequent surgical approach. In order to avoid positioning the proximal wires into the joint capsule and to reduce the risk of septic arthritis, the entrance point of the wire should be at least 14 mm distal to the joint line [115]. In 1995, Marsh et al. [116] reported 21 complex fractures of the tibial plateau in 20 patients who were treated with closed reduction, interfragmentary screw fixation of the articular fragments and application of unilateral, half-pin external fixator. Within the first 38 months, seven patients needed antibiotics for an infection at the pin site, and one had septic arthritis requiring arthrotomy and debridement [116].

In another study of 14 patients affected by high-energy atypical Schatzker type I and II fractures treated with internal fixation associated with the Ilizarov frame, five patients had minor pin track complications, and one had a superficial wound dehiscence. This combined approach has shown excellent results, without any severe soft-tissue distress, when the fracture pattern was complex [117].

The complications following tibia fractures can be divided into early (i.e. loss of reduction, deep vein thrombosis, infection) or late (i.e. non-union, malunion, implant breakage, post-traumatic arthritis, chronic infection). Early complications can be viewed as biological failures, while late complications are often associated with mechanical problems.

10.2.1 Infection

Wound-related problems are frequent and devastating complications that may lead to deep infection.

Damage to the soft-tissue envelope in the proximal tibia is frequently underestimated. Surgical incisions through bruised skin [118], with large dissection for implant positioning, often contribute to early wound breakdown and deep infection [13, 109, 119–121].

In one retrospective study of displaced tibial plateau fractures, treated with open reduction, infection occurred in 6 out of 19 AO-Muller 41. B3 (Schatzker type II) fractures (32 %) and in 7 out of 8 AO-Muller 41. B3.3 (Schatzker type IV) fractures. When fracture is complicated by infection, five, on average, subsequent surgical procedures were needed. [119].

Yang et al. [122], in a study of 44 metaphyseal dissociation fractures of the proximal tibia (Schatzker type VI) reported six deep infections (13.63 %).

Careful surgical timing, limited periosteal dissection and the reduced dissection of comminuted bone fragments are likely to decrease these complications [54, 72].

Preoperative CT scan is a very important instrument in preoperative planning, to establish the best strategy in choosing incisions and priorities, to plan the hardware (screws, plates) to be implanted, the need for bone graft, etc. Indirect reduction techniques using a femoral distractor, ligamentotaxis, percutaneous reduction clamps, small implants and percutaneously inserted can-

nulated screws further decrease the possibility of soft-tissue devascularization, wound dehiscence and deep infection [54, 123].

Twenty-four patients with Schatzker type VI tibial fractures, treated with small wire external fixation supplemented by limited internal fixation, were studied by Mikulak et al. [124] with a minimum follow-up of 12 months. There were only one septic arthritis and two infections at the screw site [124].

If wound breakdown occurs, a prompt aggressive surgical approach should be indicated. Irrigation and debridement of all devitalised and non-articular bone fragments and soft tissues are mandatory. To prevent septic arthritis and cartilage destruction, the knee joint should be thoroughly evaluated and irrigated. A deep wound infection with abscess formation should be packed open and closed secondarily, often by split-skin grafting. If a small sinus without frank pus is encountered, the wound can sometimes be closed over suction drains, after irrigation and debridement. In both scenarios, appropriate antibiotics, specific for the bacteria identified, are given intravenously for 3–6 weeks [118, 119].

The duration of antibiotic therapy must be correlated with the clinical appearance of the wound, laboratory assessment of infection parameters (erythrocyte sedimentation rate, C-reactive protein and white blood cell count) and antibiogram reports.

In the presence of infection, implants that provide stability should be retained; however, if loose, they should be removed and the fracture treated with external fixation. When the infection signs have eradicated, the fracture should be bone grafted if there is delay in healing. Revision internal fixation after sepsis requires careful judgement and great experience [118, 119].

10.2.2 Malunion and Non-union

Malunion, with late articular collapse, or deformation of the metaphysis-shaft junction, can occur after operative treatment of tibial plateau fractures [116]. A stable fixation generally reduces the incidence of these complications. If the mechanical axis is altered, an osteotomy to restore the neutral mechanical alignment is indicated. If malunion involving the articular surface occurs in an old patient, a total-knee arthroplasty may be the best salvage procedure. In some circumstances, a loss of articular reduction occurs when a major joint fragment is displaced. In these cases, early revision of the fixation should be considered, particularly if the displacement causes joint instability; late revision is extremely difficult.

Non-union is a rare complication after low-energy plateau fractures, because of the predominance of cancellous bone and the rich blood supply of the proximal tibia. It is most often seen in Schatzker type VI injuries, at the metaphyseal-diaphyseal junction. Non-union is usually the result of severe comminution, unstable fixation, unsuccessful bone grafting, mechanical failure of the implant, infection or a combination of these factors. In a study of 48 patients with 50 severe fractures of the proximal tibia treated with the use of limited internal fixation combined with external fixation and followed prospectively for 2 years, Weiner et al. [125] reported a 4 % rate of non-union requiring bone grafting. Treatment of non-union may be difficult, because of pre-existing/secondary osteoporosis, proximity to the knee joint (synovial effusion), soft-tissue scarring and prior surgical procedures.

Aseptic non-union in patients with a good bone stock should be bone grafted and the osteosynthesis should be revised, fixing the existing mechanical problems. In patients with significant osteopenia, treatment must be individualised. Internal or external fixation alone, or hybrid fixation, may be appropriate. Infected non-unions and bone deficiency require thorough early debridement of dead/infected tissue, possible implantation of antibiotic beads, free or rotational tissue flaps and external fixation.

10.3   Patella

The incidence of patella fractures has been estimated to be around 1.2 to 6.1 per 100,000 person-years [126, 127], with epidemiologic data from

Sweden, suggesting an increasing incidence in the last 30 years [128]. The risk of symptomatic hardware and knee stiffness after internal fixation is a major issue. Although hardware failure and non-union are thought to be relatively infrequent, symptomatic hardware remains a problem and often requires additional procedures [129].

Hardware removal after patella ORIF ranges from 0 to 60 % [129]. The wide variability of these reports leaves the true frequency of re-operation and complications debated. Christopher et al. [130] estimated the rate of re-operation, infection and non-union to be, respectively, 33.6 %, 3.2 % and 1.9 %. This is in accordance with data presented in a previous nonsystematic large series review [131]. It was demonstrated that age, gender, operative technique or date of publication did not significantly influence the rate of re-operation, infection or nonunion [132–137].

Other studies have shown that the incidence of non-union or delayed union of patella fractures is rare and ranges between 2.7 and 12.5 % [138]. The treatment of this complication can be challenging. The decision making is based on the functional requests of the patient, the causes of the non-union, the potential impact and the biomechanical effects of a total patellectomy, the presence of an intact extensor mechanism for subsequent reconstructive procedures.

The importance of restoring the extensor mechanism preserving the patella is well documented, and patellectomy should be reserved to limited cases.

The treatment of patella non-union and delayed union is a challenging problem with limited evidence in the literature. In addition, there are no current procedural terminology (CPT) billing codes for surgical procedures for patella non-union or delayed union. As this complication is rare, whether to preserve the entire patella or perform a patellectomy is a dilemma.

In a series of 246 fractures followed up after nonoperative treatment, Boström [139] reported no pain or discomfort in 89 % and normal or slightly impaired function in 91 % of the cases. The range of motion was 0–120° in more than 90 %. Operative management (open reduction and internal fixation, partial/total patellectomy) is the mainstay of treatment.

Preservation of the patella was described as early as 1919 [140]. The preservation of the patella is recommended in order to reduce the negative effects of patellectomy, including loss of 18° or more of knee motion, instability of the knee, 49 % reduction in the strength of the extensor mechanism and reduction in stance phase flexion excursion both in walking and stair climbing [141].

Kaufer [142] reported that after patellectomy, the knee extension requires a 30 % increase in quadriceps force. This force may be beyond the capacity of some patients, particularly those with long-lasting intra-articular disease, old age, high activity demands and an extensor mechanism deficiency before surgery. Anterior tension band wiring appears to restore excellent functional integrity in approximately 86 % of patients with very low complication rates [133, 143]. The complications most commonly reported were infection, loss of motion, hardware-related problems, refracture and delayed union or non-union.

Most patients with low functional demands with patellar non-union or delayed union are able to perform the activities of daily living with few symptoms. However, they experience difficulties in heavy work or sports activities, weakness of the affected knee. They have difficulties in climbing stairs, as they tend to adapt a gait pattern where they rotate the lower limb internally and stabilise the knee in an extended position.

The risk factors for the development of non-union or delayed union of patellar fractures are not well defined. However, some factors are more frequently associated with mal/non-consolidation, including open and transverse fractures or poor immobilisation in conservative treatment. Strong correlations exist between open fractures and the development of non-union. Torchia and Lewallen [136] reported two patients (7 %) who developed non-union among the 28 patients treated with open reduction and internal fixation for open patella fractures.

Klassen and Trousdale [138] reported 4 (21 %) open fractures out of 19 patients with patellar fractures. Open fractures of the patella occur in high-energy trauma and result in high-grade soft-tissue injury, disruption of the extensor mechanism and injury to the patellofemoral articular cartilage. Satku and Kumar [144] and Uvaraj et al. [145] noted that approximately 90 % of their patients underwent a non-surgical treatment. Inadequate immobilisation is a well-recognised cause of poor fracture healing. Information regarding the amount of initial fracture displacement was not recorded in most of the studies; therefore, the risk of non-union and delayed union relative to the amount of fracture fragment displacement could not be assessed.

Satku and Kumar [144] noted that following mobilisation and anterior tension band wiring of the fragments in patella fracture non-union, additional fixation was required. A tension loop between the proximal fragment and the tibia was used to protect the anterior tension band over the patella during knee range of motion. Two patellae out of three cases were evaluated as low-lying 2 years postoperatively. The theoretical cause of a low-lying patella (patella baja or infera) is a shortening of the patellar tendon over time which alters the biomechanics of the knee. Providing supplementation fixation in the region of the patellar tendon may act as an internal bracing during the initial rehabilitative period, but may also act as a compressive force that shortens an already reduced patellar tendon.

Klassen and Trousdale [138] reported a mean Knee Society score of 72 and function score of 78 points, with an average knee range of motion of 127° in patients with patella non-union treated conservatively. Patients treated operatively improved their mean Knee Society score from 82 to 94 points and improved their function scores from 80 to 93 points. However, the average knee motion decreased from 112° to 109°. All patients treated nonoperatively had persistent radiographic non-union signs and this was observed in only one patient of the operated group.

Uvaraj et al. [145] noted good to excellent results based on the Bostman criteria in 20 out of 22 patients treated operatively for patella fracture non-union and delayed union. Two patients had poor results due to infection, implant failure and loss of motion. The authors described difficult reductions in most of their patients. An initial cerclage wiring followed by anterior tension band wiring was helpful. The cerclage wire was removed after application of the tension band in most patients. None of the patients received quadricepsplasty for mobilisation of the fragments.

Partial or total patellectomy may be required when the patella cannot be saved. Klassen and Trousdale [138] recommended partial or total patellectomy when the fracture pattern or fragment size do not allow for internal fixation.

No specific recommendation regarding the use of bone grafts exists in literature. Klassen and Trousdale [138] reported bone grafting in two patients, but did not provide background information for their indications.

The incidence of osteoarthritis after non-union and delayed union of patella fractures is debated. Sorensen [146] noted that the risk of patellofemoral osteoarthritis was similar following nonoperative or operative fracture management. Boström [139] noted that there was no increased rate of patellofemoral osteoarthritis due to nonunion, delayed union and enlargement of the patella. The author also noted osteoarthritis was more common with an articular surface step off of 1 mm or more.

The development of osteoarthritis primarily depends on the amount of cartilage damage that occurs during the initial injury. Mehdi et al. [147], in a series of 203 cases of patella fracture treated with tension band wiring, reported that 17 out of 203 patients (8.5 %) developed patellofemoral arthritis.

Non-union and delayed union of fractures of the patella are uncommon. However, open fractures, improper immobilisation and the initial fracture configuration should raise the surgeon's vigilance. Patients with low functional demands may be managed with nonoperative methods; on the other hand, patients involved in heavy physical work or sports usually require open reduction and internal fixation. Operative management appears to play a major role in restoring the functional integrity of the extensor mechanism. Tension band wiring is the treatment of choice for patients suitable for a reconstructive procedure. Partial or total patellectomy is also an option for small distal fragments or when satisfactory internal fixation cannot be achieved. Regarding the management of non-union and delayed union following patella fractures, prospective, randomised, multicentre studies are needed to develop evidence-based recommendations (Figs. 10.1, 10.2, 10.3, 10.4, and 10.5).

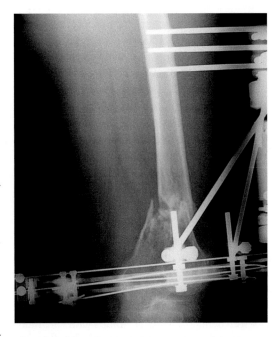

Fig. 10.1 Male, 53 years old at the time of the trauma, obese, diabetes mellitus, hardworker. Patient was referred to our institution from a suburban hospital for a left sacroiliac dissociation 1 month after an MVA. Coexisting left open distal femur fracture, AO 33.C1, treated initially by means of closed reduction and hybrid external fixator. The knee ROM was about 40°-10°-10°

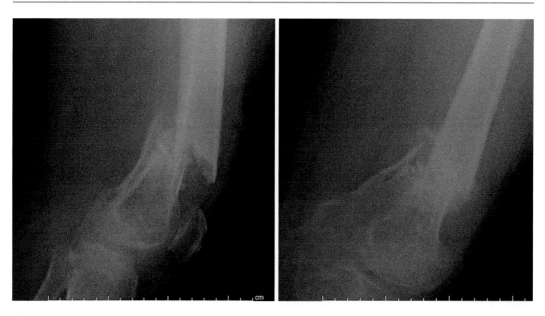

Fig. 10.2 Six months after the trauma, no signs of radiological healing, the fracture site was still unstable. The frame was removed, the patient was put in a splint for 45 days in order to achieve wound healing

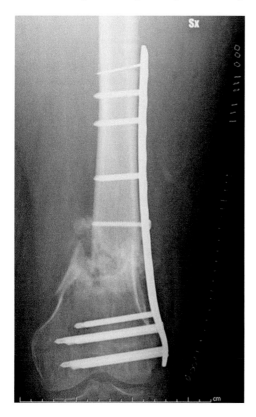

Fig. 10.3 Post-op x-ray after non-union site debridement, open reduction, fixation with an LCP-LISS 4.5 plate in compression. At the same time extra-articular arthrolysis getting a satisfactory ROM in the operating room (130°-5°-5°). Full weight bearing was allowed 2 days after surgery (after drain removal)

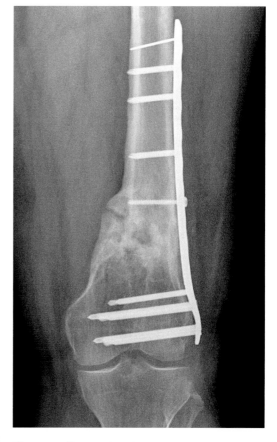

Fig. 10.4 Six months after non-union revision. The patient was walking with no crutches, no pain, ROM 100°-5°-5°, very mild limping

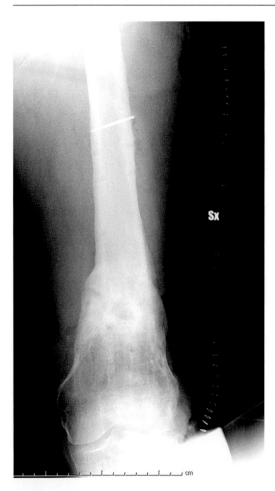

Fig. 10.5 Fifteen months after non-union surgery. Plate removal, in the operating room, the callus appeared to be completely healed. The patient was walking with no crutches, no pain, ROM 100°-5°-5°, no limping

References

1. Watson-Jones R (1957) Fractures and joint injuries. Williams & Wilkins, Baltimore
2. Bolhofner BR, Carmen B, Clifford P (1996) The results of open reduction and internal fixation of distal femur fractures using a biologic (indirect) reduction technique. J Orthop Trauma 10:372–377
3. Henry SL, Trager S, Green S et al (1991) Management of supracondylar fractures of the femur with the GSH intramedullary nail: preliminary report. Contemp Orthop 22:631–640
4. Tscherne H (1991) Femoral shaft and distal femur. In: Muller ME, Allgower M, Schneider R et al (eds) Manual of internal fixation. Springer, Berlin, pp 548–552
5. Benum P (1977) The use of bone cement as an adjunct to internal fixation of supracondylar fractures of osteoporotic femurs. Acta Orthop Scand 48:52–56
6. Chiron HS, Tremoulet J, Casey P et al (1974) Fractures of the distal third of the femur treated by internal fixation. Clin Orthop 100:160–170
7. Connolly JF, Dehne E, Lafollette B (1973) Closed reduction and early cast-brace ambulation in the treatment of femoral fractures: II. Results in one hundred and forty-three fractures. J Bone Joint Surg Am 55:1581–1599
8. Connolly JF, King P (1973) Closed reduction and early cast-brace ambulation in the treatment of femoral fractures: I. An in vivo quantitative analysis of immobilization in skeletal traction and a cast brace. J Bone Joint Surg Am 55:1559–1580
9. Halpenny J, Rorabeck CH (1984) Supracondylar fractures of the femur: results of treatment of sixty-one patients. Can J Surg 27:606–609
10. Healy WL, Brooker AFJ (1983) Distal femoral fractures: comparison of open and closed methods of treatment. Clin Orthop 174:166–171
11. Mooney V, Nickel VL, Harvey JPJ et al (1970) Cast-brace treatment of fractures of the distal part of the femur: a prospective controlled study of one hundred and fifty patients. J Bone Joint Surg Am 52:1563–1578
12. Neer CS, Grantham SA, Shelton ML (1967) Supracondylar fracture of the adult femur: a study of one hundred and ten cases. J Bone Joint Surg Am 49:591–613
13. Schatzker J, Home G, Waddell J (1974) The Toronto experience with the supracondylar fracture of the femur, 1966–72. Injury 6:113–128
14. Schatzker J, Lambert DC (1979) Supracondylar fractures of the femur. Clin Orthop 138:77–83
15. Scuderi C, Ippolito A (1952) Nonunion of supracondylar fractures of the femur. J Int Coll Surg 17:1–18
16. Seinsheimer F (1980) Fractures of the distal femur. Clin Orthop 169–179
17. Slatis P, Ryoppy S, Huittinen VM (1971) AOI osteosynthesis of fractures of the distal third of the femur. Acta Orthop Scand 42:162–172
18. Stewart MJ, Sisk TD, Wallace SL (1966) Fractures of the distal third of the femur: a comparison of methods of treatment. J Bone Joint Surg Am 48:784–807
19. Weil GC, Kuehner HG, Henry JP (1936) The treatment of 278 consecutive fractures of the femur. Surg Gynecol Obstet 62:435–441
20. Funsten RV, Lee RW (1945) Healing time in fracture of the shafts of the tibia and femur. J Bone Joint Surg Am 27:395–400
21. Kessler SB, Hallfeldt KK, Perren SM et al (1986) The effects of reaming and intramedullary nailing on fracture healing. Clin Orthop 212:18–25
22. Schandelmaier P, Partenhemer A, Koanemann B et al (2001) Distal femoral fractures and LISS stabilisation. Injury 32:SC 55–63
23. Kanabar P, Kumar V, Owen PJ, Rushton N (2007) Less invasive stabilisation system plating for distal femoral fractures. J Orthop Surg 15:299–302

24. Schatzker J (1998) Fractures of the distal femur revisited. Clin Orthop Relat Res 347:43–56
25. Apostolou CD, Papavasiliou AV, Aslam N et al (2005) Preliminary results and technical aspects following stabilisation of fractures around the knee with liss. Injury 36:529–36
26. Syed AA, Agarwal M, Giannoudis PV et al (2004) Distal femoral fractures: long-term outcome following stabilisation with the LISS. Injury 35:599–607
27. Wiss D, Watson J, Johnson E (1996) Fractures of the knee. In: Rockwood CA, Green DP, Bucholz RW et al (eds) Rockwood and Green's fractures in adults. Lippincott-Raven, Philadelphia, pp 1919–99
28. Mize RD, Bucholz RW, Grogan DP (1982) Surgical treatment of displaced, comminuted fractures of the distal end of the femur. J Bone Joint Surg 64A:871
29. Ali F, Saleh M (2000) Treatment of isolated complex distal femoral fractures by external fixation. Injury 31(3):139–46
30. Danziger MB, Caucei D, Zecher SB, Segal D, Covall DJ (1995) Treatment of intercondylar and supracondylar distal femoral fractures using the GSH supracondylar nail. Am J Orthop 24(9):684–90
31. Zickel RE (1988) Non-union of fractures of the proximal and distal thirds of the shaft of the femur. Instruct Course Lect 37:173–9
32. Altenberg AR, Shorkey RL (1949) Blade plate fixation in non-union and complicated fractures of the supracondylar region of the femur. J Bone Joint Surg 31A:312–6
33. Chapman MW, Finkemeiere CG (1999) Treatment of supracondylar nonunions of the femur with plate fixation and bone graft. J Bone Joint Surg 81A:1217–28
34. Bellabarba C, Ricci WM, Bolhofner BR (2002) Indirect reduction and plating of distal femoral nonunions. J Orthop Trauma 16:287–296
35. Haidukewych GJ, Berry DJ, Jacofsky DJ, Torchia ME (2003) Treatment of supracondylar femur nonunions with open reduction and internal fixation. Am J Orthop 32:564–567
36. Wang JW, Weng LH (2003) Treatment of distal femoral nonunion with internal fixation, cortical allograft struts, and autogenous bonegrafting. J Bone Joint Surg Am 85-A:436–440
37. Wu CC, Shih CH (1995) Distal femoral non-union treated with interlocking nailing. J Trauma 31(12):1659–62
38. Mc Laren AC, Blokker CP (1991) Locked intramedullary fixation for metaphyseal malunion and non-union. Clin Orthop 265:253–60
39. Kempf I, Grosse A, Rigaut P (1986) The treatment of noninfected pseudo-arthrosis of the femur and tibia with locked intramedullary nailing. Clin Orthop 212:142–54
40. Koval KJ, Seligson D, Rosen H, Fee K (1995) Distal femoral nonunion: treatment with a retrograde-inserted locked intramedullary nail. J Orthop Trauma 9(4):285–91
41. Beall MS, Nebel E, Bailey RW (1979) Transarticular fixation is the treatment of non-union of supra-condylar fractures of the femur: a salvage procedure. J Bone Joint Surg 61A:1018–23
42. Moore TJ, Watson T, Green SA et al (1987) Complications of surgically treated supracondylar fractures of the femur. J Trauma 27(4):402–6
43. Marsh JL, Nepola JV, Meffert R (1992) Dynamic external fixation for stabilisation of nonunions. Clin Orthop 278:200–6
44. Di Pasquale D, Gage Ochsner M, Kelly AM, Murphy MD (1994) The Ilizarov method for complex fracture nonunions. J Trauma 37(4):629–34
45. Catagni M (1991) Classification and treatment of nonunions. In: Maiocchi AB, Aronson J (eds) Operative principles of Ilizarov. Williams and Wilkins, Baltimore
46. Mandt PR, Gershuni DH (1987) Treatment of non-union of fractures in the epiphyseal–metaphyseal region of long bones. J Orthop Trauma 1(2):141–51
47. Charnley J, Baker SL (1952) Compression arthrodesis of the knee. A clinical and histological study. J Bone Joint Surg 34B:187–99
48. Zum Brunnen C, Brindley H (1968) Nonunion of long bones. Analysis of 144 cases. J Am Med Assoc 203:637
49. Saleh M (1992) Non-union surgery Part I. Basic principles of management. Intl J Orthop Trauma 2:4–18
50. Freedman EL, Hak DJ, Johnson EE et al (1995) Total knee replacement including a modular distal femoral component in elderly patients with acute fracture or nonunion. J Orthop Trauma 9:231–237
51. Olerud S (1972) Operative treatment of supracondylar–condylar fractures of the femur: technique and results in fifteen cases. J Bone Joint Surg Am 54:1015–1032
52. Mahorner HR, Bradburn M (1933) Fractures of the femur: report of three hundred and eight cases. Surg Gynecol Obstet 56:1066–1079
53. Kinast C, Bolhofner BR, Mast JW et al (1989) Subtrochanteric fractures of the femur: results of treatment with the ninety-five degrees condylar blade-plate. Clin Orthop 238:122–130
54. Mast J, Jakob R, Ganz R (1989) Planning and reduction technique in fracture surgery. Springer, Berlin
55. Pritchett JW (1984) Supracondylar fractures of the femur. Clin Orthop 184:173–177
56. Rosen H (1979) Compression treatment of long bone pseudarthroses. Clin Orthop 138:154–166
57. Cove JA, Lhowe DW, Jupiter JB et al (1997) The management of femoral diaphyseal nonunions. J Orthop Trauma 11:513–520
58. McLaren AC, Blokker CP (1991) Locked intramedullary fixation for metaphyseal malunion and non-union. Clin Orthop 265:253–260
59. Shahcheraghi GH, Doroodchi HR (1993) Supracondylar fracture of the femur: closed or open reduction? J Trauma 34:499–502
60. Solheim K, Vaage S (1973) Delayed union and non-union of fractures: clinical experience with the ASIF method. J Trauma 13:121–128

61. Tarr RR, Wiss DA (1986) The mechanics and biology of intramedullary fracture fixation. Clin Orthop 212:10–17

62. Fankhauser F, Gruber G, Schippinger G et al (2004) Minimal-invasive treatment of distal femoral fractures with the LISS (less invasive stabilization system). Acta Orthop Scand 75:56–60

63. Frigg R, Appenzeller A, Christensen R et al (2001) The development of the distal femur less invasive stabilization system (LISS). Injury 32:SC 24–31

64. Muller ME, Allgower M, Schneider R, Willenegger H (1990) Manual of Internal fixation. Techniques reommended by the AOASIF Group. Springer, New York

65. Marti A, Fankhauser C, Frenk A et al (2001) Biomechanical evaluation of the less invasive stabilization system for the internal fixation of distal femur fractures. J Orthop Trauma 15:482

66. Bong MR, Egol KA, Koval KJ et al (2002) Comparison of the LISS and a retrograde inserted supracondylar intramedullary nail for fixation of a periprosthetic distal femur fracture proximal to a total knee arthroplasty. J Arthroplasty 17:876–81

67. Zlowodzki M, Williamson S, Cole PA et al (2004) Biomechanical evaluation of the less invasive stabilization system, angled blade plate, and retrograde intramedullary nail for the internal fixation of distal femur fractures. J Orthop Trauma 18:494–502

68. Karnezis IA, Miles AW, Cunningham JL, Learmonth ID (1998) "Biological" internal fixation of long bone fractures: a biomechanical study of a "noncontact" plate system. Injury 29(9):689–695

69. Schutz M, Sudkamp NP (2003) Revolution in plate osteosynthesis: new internal fixator systems. J Orthop Sci 8(2):252–258

70. Marsh DR, Shah S, Elliott J et al (1997) The Ilizarov method in nonunion, malunion and infection of fractures. J Bone Joint Surg Br 79:273–279

71. Siliski JM, Mahring M, Hofer HP (1989) Supracondylar-intercondylar fractures of the femur: treatment by internal fixation. J Bone Joint Surg Am 71:95–104

72. Mast JW, Teitge RA, Gowda M (1990) Preoperative planning for the treatment of nonunions and the correction of malunions of the long bones. Orthop Clin North Am 21:693–714

73. Ali F, Saleh M (2002) Treatment of distal femoral non-unions by external fixation with simultaneous length and alignment correction. Injury 33:127–34

74. Johnson KD, Hicken G (1987) Distal femoral fractures. Orthop Clin North Am 18:115–32

75. Webb LX (2001) Bone defect non-union of the lower extremity. Tech Orthop 164:387–97

76. Ilizarov GA (1992) Transosseous osteosynthesis. Theoretical and clinical aspects of the regeneration and growth of tissue. Springer, Berlin

77. Ilizarov GA (1971) Osnovnye printsipy chreskostnogo kompressionnogo i distraktsionnogo osteosinteza. Orthop Traumatol Protez 32:7–15

78. Ilizarov GA (1989) Fractures and nonunions. In: Coombs R, Green S, Sarmiento A (eds) External fixation and functional bracing. Aspen, London, pp 347–357

79. Ilizarov GA (1989) Fractures and nonunions. In: Coombs R, Green S, Sarmiento A (eds) External fixation and functional bracing. Aspen, London, pp 249–281

80. Ilizarov GA (1989) The tension-stress effect on the genesis and growth of tissues: I. The influence of stability of fixation and soft-tissue preservation. Clin Orthop 238:249–281

81. Ilizarov GA (1989) The tension-stress effect on the genesis and growth of tissues: II. The influence of the rate and frequency of distraction. Clin Orthop 238:263–285

82. Paley D, Chaudray M, Pirone AM et al (1990) Treatment of malunions and mal-nonunions of the femur and tibia by detailed preoperative planning and the Ilizarov techniques. Orthop Clin North Am 21:667–691

83. Saleh M, Royston S (1996) Management of nonunion of fractures by distraction with correction of angulation and shortening. J Bone Joint Surg Br 78:105–109

84. Association for the Study and Application of the Method of Ilizarov Group: non-union of the femur (1991) In: Bianchi-Maiocchi A, Aronson J (eds) Operative principles of Ilizarov. Fracture treatment, non-union, osteomyelitis, lengthening, deformity correction. Williams and Wilkins, Baltimore

85. Aronson J, Johnson E, Harp JH (1989) Local bone transportation for treatment of intercalary defects by the Ilizarov technique. Biomechanical and clinical considerations. Clin Orthop Relat Res 243:71–9

86. Cattaneo R, Catagni M, Johnson EE (1992) The treatment of infected nonunions and segmented defects of the tibia by the methods of Ilizarov. Clin Orthop Relat Res 280:143–52

87. Dendrinos GK, Kontos S, Lyritsis E (1995) Use of the Ilizarov technique for treatment of non-union of the tibia associated with infection. J Bone Joint Surg Am 77:835–46

88. Song HR, Kale A, Park HB, Koo KH, Chae DJ, Oh CW et al (2003) Comparison of internal bone transport and vascularized fibular grafting for femoral bone defects. J Orthop Trauma 17:203–11

89. Barbarossa V, Matkovic BR, Vucic N, Bielen M, Gluhinic M (2001) Treatment of osteomyelitis and infected non-union of the femur by a modified Ilizarov technique: follow-up study. Croat Med J 42:634–41

90. Gualdrini G, Stagni C, Fravisini M, Giunti A (2002) Infected nonunion of the femur. Chir Organ Mov 87:225–33

91. Paley D (1990) Problems, obstacles, and complications of limb lengthening by the Ilizarov technique. Clin Orthop Relat Res 250:81–104

92. Theis JC, Simpson H, Kenwright J (2000) Correction of complex lower limb deformities by the Ilizarov

technique: an audit of complications. J Orthop Surg (Hong Kong) 8:67–71

93. Shevtsov V, Popkov A, Popkov D, Prevot J (2001) Reduction of the period of treatment for leg lengthening. Technique and advantages [in French]. Rev Chir Orthop Reparatrice Appar Mot 87:248–56

94. Conway JD, Mont MA, Bezwada HP (2004) Arthrodesis of the knee. J Bone Joint Surg Am A 86:835–48

95. Waters RL, Perry J, Antonelli D, Hislop H (1976) Energy cost of walking of amputees: the influence of the level of amputation. J Bone Joint Surg Am 58:42–6

96. Tokizaki T, Abe S, Tateishi A, Hirose M, Matsushita T (2004) Distraction osteogenesis for knee arthrodesis in infected tumour prostheses. Clin Orthop Relat Res 424:166–72

97. De Pablos J, Barrios C, Canadell J (1991) Leg lengthening by distraction through the callus of an arthrodesis. J Bone Joint Surg Br 73:458–60

98. Rozbruch SR, Ilizarov S, Blyakher A (2005) Knee arthrodesis with simultaneous lengthening using the Ilizarov method. J Orthop Trauma 19:171–9

99. Rand JA (1993) Alternatives to reimplantation for salvage of the total knee arthroplasty complicated by infection. J Bone Joint Surg Am 75:282–9

100. Vlasak R, Gearen PF, Petty W (1995) Knee arthrodesis in the treatment of failed total knee replacement. Clin Orthop Relat Res 321:138–44

101. Salem K, Kinzl L, Schmelz A (2006) Circular external fixation in knee arthrodesis following septic trauma sequelae. J Knee Surg 19:99–104

102. Kinik H (2009) Knee arthrodesis with Ilizarov's bone transport method for large infected periarticular defects: a report of three cases. J Trauma 67:E213–9

103. Lansinger O, Bergman B, Korner L, Andersson GB (1986) Tibial condylar fractures. A twenty-year follow-up. J Bone Joint Surg Am 68(1):13–9

104. Rasmussen PS (1973) Tibial condylar fractures. Impairment of knee joint stability as an indicator for surgical treatment. J Bone Joint Surg Am 55(7):1331–50

105. Behrens FF (1993) Knee and leg, bone trauma. In: Frymoyer J (ed) Orthopaedic knowledge update-4. Academy of Orthopaedic Surgeons, Rosemont, pp 579–92

106. Decoster TA, Nepola JV, el-Khoury GY (1988) Cast brace treatment of proximal tibial plateau fractures. Ten year follow-up study. Clin Orthop 231:196–204

107. Behrens FF (1989) General theory and principles of external fixation. Clin Orthop 241:15–23

108. Wyrsch B, McFerran MA, McAndrew M et al (1996) Operative treatment of fractures of the tibial plateau. A randomized, prospective study. J Bone Joint Surg Am 78(11):1646–57

109. Wadell AP, Johnston DWC, Meidre A (1981) Fractures of tibial plateau, a review of 95 patients and comparison of treatment methods. J Trauma 2:376–81

110. Muller ME, Allgower M, Schneider R, Willenegger H (1992) Manual der Osteosynthese. Springer, New York/Berlin/Heidelberg

111. Tscherne H, Lobenhoffer P (1993) Tibial plateau fractures, management and expected results. Clin Orthop 292:87–100

112. Lachiewicz PF, Funcik T (1990) Factors influencing the results of open reduction and internal fixation of tibial plateau fractures. Clin Orthop 259:210–5

113. Dendrinos GK, Kontos S, Katsenis D, Dalas A (1996) Treatment of high-energy tibial plateau fractures by the Ilizarov Circular Fixator. J Bone Joint Surg Br 78(5):710–7

114. Harwood PJ, Giannoudis PV, Probst C, Krettek C, Pape HC (2006) The risk of local infective complications after damage control procedures for femoral shaft fracture. J Orthop Trauma 20(3):181–9

115. Reid JS, Van Slyke MA, Moulton MJ, Mann TA (2001) Safe placement of proximal tibial transfixation wires with respect to intracapsular penetration. J Orthop Trauma 15(1):10–7

116. Marsh JL, Smith ST, Do TT (1995) External fixation and limited internal fixation for complex fractures of the tibial plateau. J Bone Joint Surg Am 77(5):661–73

117. Watson JT, Coufal C (1998) Treatment of complex lateral plateau fractures using Ilizarov techniques. Clin Orthop 353:97–106

118. Oestern HJ, Tscherne H (1983) Pathophysiology and classification of soft tissue damage in fractures. Orthopade 12(1):2–8

119. Young MJ, Barrack RL (1994) Complications of internal fixation of tibial plateau fractures. Orthop Rev 23:149–54

120. Fernandez DL (1988) Anterior approach to the knee with osteotomy of the tibial tubercle for bicondylar tibial plateau fractures. J Bone Joint Surg Am 70(2):208–19

121. Mallik AR, Covall DJ, Whitelaw GP (1992) Internal versus external fixation of bicondylar tibial plateau fractures. Orthop Rev 21(12):1433–6

122. Yang EC, Weiner L, Strauss E et al (1995) Metaphyseal dissociation fractures of the proximal tibia. An analysis of treatment and complications. Am J Orthop 244:695–704

123. Muller ME, Nazarian S, Koch P et al (1990) The comprehensive classification of fractures and long bones. Springer, New York

124. Mikulak SA, Gold SM, Zinar DM (1998) Small wire external fixation of high energy tibial plateau fractures. Clin Orthop 356:230–8

125. Weiner LS, Kelley M, Yang E et al (1995) The use of combination internal fixation and hybrid external fixation in severe proximal tibia fractures. J Orthop Trauma 9(3):244–50

126. van Staa TP, Dennison EM, Leufkens HG, Cooper C (2001) Epidemiology of fractures in England and Wales. Bone 29:517–522

127. Yang NP, Chan CL, Yu IL, Lee CY, Chou P (2010) Estimated prevalence of orthopaedic fractures in

Taiwan Va cross-sectional study based on nationwide insurance data. Injury 41:1266–1272

128. Bengner U, Johnell O, Redlund-Johnell I (1986) Increasing incidence of tibia condyle and patella fractures. Acta Orthop Scand 57:334–336

129. Melvin JS, Mehta S (2011) Patellar fractures in adults. J Am Acad Orthop Surg 19:198–207

130. Dy CJ, Little MT, Berkes MB, Ma Y, Roberts TR, Helfet DL, Lorich DG (2012) Meta-analysis of re-operation, nonunion, and infection after open reduction and internal fixation of patella fractures. J Trauma Acute Care Surg 73(4):928–32

131. Warriner AH, Patkar NM, Curtis JR, et al (2011) Which fractures are most attributable to osteoporosis? J Clin Epidemiol 64:46–53

132. Bostman O, Kiviluoto O, Nirhamo J (1981) Comminuted displaced fractures of the patella. Injury 13:196–202

133. Bostman O, Kiviluoto O, Santavirta S, Nirhamo J, Wilppula E (1983) Fractures of the patella treated by operation. Arch Orthop Trauma Surg 102:78–81

134. Hung LK, Chan KM, Chow YN, Leung PC (1985) Fractured patella: operative treatment using the tension band principle. Injury 16:343–347

135. Wu CC, Tai CL, Chen WJ (2001) Patellar tension band wiring: a revised technique. Arch Orthop Trauma Surg 121:12–16

136. Torchia ME, Lewallen DG (1996) Open fractures of the patella. J Orthop Trauma 10:403–409

137. Saltzman CL, Goulet JA, McClellan RT, Schneider LA, Matthews LS (1990) Results of treatment of displaced patellar fractures by partial patellectomy. J Bone Joint Surg Am 72:1279–1285

138. Klassen JF, Trousdale RT (1997) Treatment of delayed and nonunion of the patella. J Orthop Trauma 11(3):188–194

139. Boström A (1974) Longitudinal fractures of the patella. Reconstr Surg Traumatol 14:136–146

140. Albee FH (1919) Ununited fracture of the patella and of the olecranon. Surg Gynecol Obstet 28:422

141. Sutton FS Jr, Thompson CH, Lipke J, Kettelkamp DB (1976) The effect of patellectomy on knee function. J Bone Joint Surg Am 58(4):537–540

142. Kaufer H (1971) Mechanical function of the patella. J Bone Joint Surg Am 53(8):1551–1560

143. Nummi J (1971) Operative treatment of patellar fractures. Acta Orthop Scand 42(5):437–438

144. Satku K, Kumar VP (1991) Surgical management of non-union of neglected fractures of the patella. Injury 22(2):108–110

145. Uvaraj NR, Mayil Vahanan N, Sivaseelam A, Mohd Sameer M, Basha IM (2007) Surgical management of neglected fractures of the patella. Injury 38(8):979–983

146. Sorensen KH (1964) The late prognosis after fracture of the patella. Acta Orthop Scand 34:198–212

147. Mehdi M, Husson JL, Polard JL, Ouahmed A, Poncher R, Lombard J (1999) Treatment results of fractures of the patella using pre-patellar tension wiring. Analysis of a series of 203 cases (in French). Acta Orthop Belg 65(2):188–196

Management of the Complications Following Fractures Around the Knee (Malalignment and Unicompartmental Arthritis)

11

Davide Edoardo Bonasia, Filippo Castoldi, Massimiliano Dragoni, and Annunziato Amendola

11.1 Introduction

The treatment of diffuse or unicompartmental knee arthrosis in the young patient is still a challenge for the orthopedic surgeon. The ideal management should resolve the pain, restore the function, and preserve the anatomy without jeopardizing, if necessary, an eventual subsequent total joint replacement. The goal of this chapter is to discuss the range of possible treatments for patellofemoral (PF) and femorotibial post-traumatic arthrosis, when the degeneration is too severe to perform cartilage resurfacing procedures and the patient is too young and active to undergo a total joint replacement.

11.2 Patellofemoral Joint

11.2.1 Clinical Examination

The history of patients with post-traumatic PF arthrosis should be thoroughly evaluated, with particular attention to the traumatic mechanism, previous reduction and fixation procedure, patellar dislocation, residual instability, and previous additional procedures (arthroscopic debridement, microfractures, lateral release, and extensor mechanism realignment). Patients typically report pain during flexed knee activities that increase PF pressure, and these include (1) squatting, (2) prolonged seated position, (3) going up, and, more commonly, downstairs. The physical examination should commence with an assessment of the whole lower limb, with particular attention to axial and rotational deformities. The range of motion (ROM) of the knee should be evaluated together with the patellar tracking. Evaluation of medial

D.E. Bonasia MD (✉)
University of Torino, AO Mauriziano
"Umberto I" Hospital, Via Lamarmora 26,
Torino 10128, Italy
e-mail: davidebonasia@virgilio.it

F. Castoldi
University of Torino, AO Città della
Salute e della Scienza di Torino,
CTO Hospital, Turin, Italy
e-mail: filippo.castoldi@unito.it

M. Dragoni
University of Tor Vergata, Rome, Italy
e-mail: massi.dragoni@gmail.com

A. Amendola
Department of Orthopaedics and Rehabilitation,
University of Iowa Sports Medicine,
University of Iowa, Iowa city,
IA 52242, USA
e-mail: ned-amendola@uiowa.edu

© Springer International Publishing Switzerland 2016
F. Castoldi, D.E. Bonasia (eds.), *Fractures Around the Knee*, Fracture Management Joint by Joint,
DOI 10.1007/978-3-319-28806-2_11

and lateral patellar displacement, patellar tilt, and focal areas of pain is essential. The Q angle is the angle formed by a line drawn from the anterosuperior iliac spine (ASIS) to the center of the patella and a second line drawn from the center of the patella to the tibial tubercle; the Q angle can be measured clinically or radiographically on long leg X-rays. The normal values are 14 deg (+/− 3) for males and 17 deg (+/− 3) for females [1].

11.2.2 Imaging and Preoperative Workup

Radiographically, anteroposterior, true lateral, Rosenberg, and axial (Merchant or skyline) views are required for a correct evaluation of the PF joint. Hip-to-ankle single weight-bearing radiographs may be required to evaluate lower limb axial deformities. Traditional radiographs are useful to determine the severity of arthritic degeneration, possible patellar tilts, Q angle (long leg X-rays), patellar height (Insall-Salvati, Caton-Deschamps, or Blackburne-Peel indices), and trochlear dysplasia (crossing sign, double contour, and anterior spur evident on true lateral views of the knee).

Computed tomography (CT) and magnetic resonance imaging (MRI) are often required to complete PF joint evaluation. CT has been considered for more than 20 years as the gold standard for measuring the tibial tuberosity-trochlear groove distance (TT-GT), the tilt angle, the sulcus angle, and the congruence angle and for studying the anatomy of the patella and trochlea. CT is the gold standard also for the quantification of torsional defects of the lower limb (most of all femoral antiversion, but also tibial external rotation), which may considerably affect PF tracking, predisposing to instability. For this purpose, with the patient supine and the feet 15° externally rotated, sections are obtained at the level of the femoral neck, PF joint, tibial tubercle, and ankle joint.

Dynamic CT scan with the quadriceps contracted at different degrees of knee flexion may be useful to precisely assess the patellar tracking, when the clinical examination is not sufficient.

Recently, many authors expanded the indications of MRI to include different measurements (TT-GT distance, tilt angle, sulcus angle, and congruence angle) besides the articular cartilage and soft tissue evaluation.

The TT-GT measures the distance between the deepest part of the trochlear groove and the tibial tubercle. Normal values range from 10 to 15 mm [2]. When the value is >15 mm lateral, PF excessive pressure syndrome is usually present, and distal extensor mechanism realignment may be considered alone or combined with other procedures.

11.2.3 Classification

Since osteochondral defects are not one of the goals of this chapter, any classification system for knee arthrosis may be used. Merchant et al. [3] specifically staged the severity of PF disease based on the 45° skyline view as stage zero is normal; stage one is mild with more than 3-mm joint space; stage two is moderate with less than 3-mm joint space but no bony contact; stage three is severe with bony surfaces in contact over less than one quarter of the joint surface; and stage four is very severe with bony contact throughout the joint surfaces.

11.2.4 Indications

The treatment of isolated post-traumatic PF joint arthrosis is challenging, and no decision-making algorithms are available in the English literature. The treatments described for this condition include (1) conservative management, (2) cheiloplasty or facetectomy (with or without lateral release or medial plication), (3) patellectomy, (4) tibial tubercle osteotomy, (5) PF joint replacement, and

(6) total joint replacement. Cartilage resurfacing alone or with realignment procedures is indicated in young patients with focal defects, but this is not the focus of this chapter.

11.2.4.1   Conservative Treatment

Conservative treatment is mainly focused on (1) intra-articular injections (corticosteroids or viscosupplementation), (2) core and strengthening of the thigh muscles, (3) bracing, (4) weight loss, and (5) nonsteroidal anti-inflammatory drugs (NSAIDs).

11.2.4.2   Lateral Retinacular Release

In patients with early lateral PF arthritis, lateral release may be considered. This may relieve the symptoms of pain, but does not always result in a normal patellar alignment. If there are overhanging lateral osteophytes, these can be removed at the same time arthroscopically or with open technique, if an extracapsular lateral release is preferred [4].

11.2.4.3   Patellectomy

Even though the results reported for patellectomy appear controversial, patellar removal undoubtedly reduces extensor mechanism function and affects the functional outcomes of any later total knee replacement (TKR) [4]. In our view, patellectomy should be avoided if possible and reserved to those patients who are not candidate to any resurfacing or replacement procedure (i.e., active infection, severe posttraumatic abnormalities of the extensor mechanism, etc.).

11.2.4.4   Tibial Tubercle Osteotomy

Tibial tubercle osteotomy was popularized by Maquet (anterior displacement) and Elmslie-Trillat (medial displacement), and good results were reported in terms of realignment [2]. Nevertheless, the functional outcomes in PF arthrosis were reported to be satisfactory in 65–80 % of the patients [4]. Although little independent literature is present about Fulkerson's procedure (anteromedial displacement), this technique seems to produce good results in early PF arthrosis. This technique can be performed alone in case of early lateral PF arthrosis due to malalignment or combined with PF arthroplasty in case of severe articular degeneration and patellar maltracking (Figs. 11.1 and 11.2).

11.2.4.5   Patellofemoral Arthroplasty

Patellofemoral arthroplasty (PFA), first attempted in the 1970s, recently rose in popularity for the treatment of isolated PF arthrosis in the young patient. PFA indications include (1) severe PF

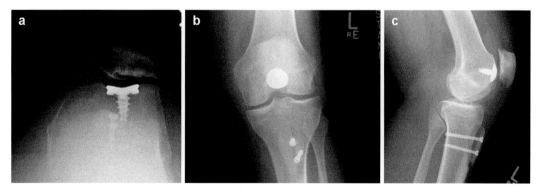

Fig. 11.1 Isolated initial PF arthrosis with malalignment. (**a–c**) Postoperative skyline, anteroposterior, and lateral views of the knee, after minimally invasive PF arthroplasty and Fulkerson's distal realignment

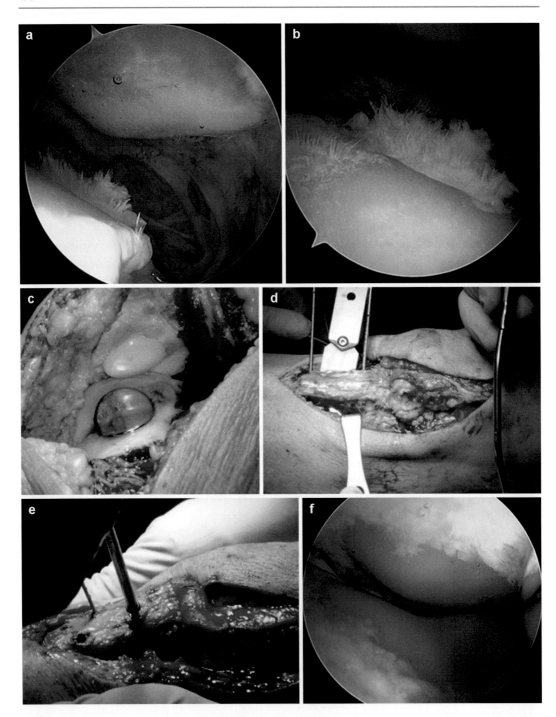

Fig. 11.2 Intraoperative pictures of the case described in Fig. 11.1. (**a, b**) Arthroscopic evidence of bone-on-bone PF arthrosis. (**c**) Component positioning. (**d, e**) Fulkerson's distal realignment and fixation of the tubercle osteotomy with 2 cortical screws. (**f**) Arthroscopy performed 18 months later for other reasons, showing good PF tracking and alignment

arthrosis; (2) failure of conservative treatment (for at least 6 months); (3) absence of symptomatic tibiofemoral arthrosis; (4) absence of malalignment (or when malalignment has been corrected); (5) intact surrounding menisci, cruciate, and collateral ligaments; and (6) patients older than 40 years old. Many implants with different features are available on the market. These can be mainly divided in three types: (1) inlay implants (the trochlear component surface is at the same level of the surrounding articular surface); (2) onlay implants (the trochlear component surface is prominent compared to the surrounding articular surface) (Figs. 11.3 and 11.4); and (3) minimally invasive implants (with minimal cartilage/bone resection and component implantation with inlay technique) (Figs. 11.1 and 11.2).

11.2.4.6   Minimally Invasive Patellofemoral Implants

Minimally invasive PFAs have been recently introduced (Figs. 11.1 and 11.2). The goal of these implants is to replace only the degenerated area of the PF joint with inlay components that require minimal bone resection, preserving the bone stock for and easier subsequent TKR [5]. However, these implants are rarely used in post-traumatic PF arthrosis, due to the diffuse degeneration of the joint, requiring larger arthroplasties.

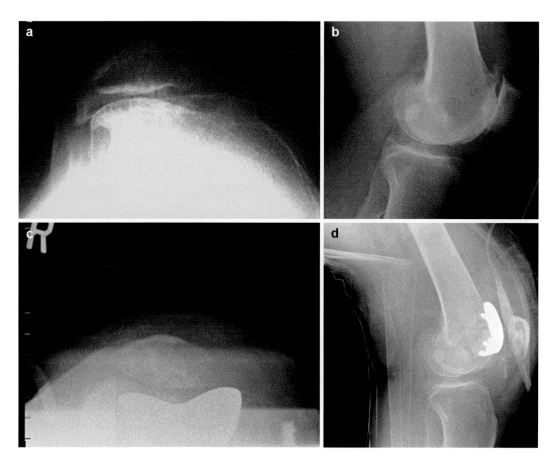

Fig. 11.3 Isolated severe PF arthrosis. (**a, b**) Preoperative skyline and lateral views of the knee. (**c, d**) Postoperative skyline and lateral views of the knee, after formal PF replacement

11.2.5 Surgical Techniques

11.2.5.1 Tibial Tuberosity Osteotomy

In the Fulkerson's procedure, a 5–6 cm anterior incision slightly lateral to the tibial tuberosity is performed, starting at the level of the joint line and prolonged distally. If combined lateral release is planned, this can be either done arthroscopically or open (extending the incision proximally). The tibialis anterior is elevated from the lateral surface of the tibia with a Cobb elevator. The medial and lateral borders of the patellar tendon and tuberosity are carefully delineated. The periosteum along the medial side of the tuberosity is incised 5–8 cm distal to the tuberosity. Distally, the osteotomy should narrow and taper, allowing it to act as a hinge. One or two 1.5-mm K wires are inserted from the anteromedial aspect of the tuberosity to the posterolateral aspect, with an inclination of about 30°. The osteotomy is performed (anterior with respect to the K wires) with a thin oscillating saw and completed with osteotomies. Once the osteotomy is completed proximally and preserving the distal hinge, the tibial tuberosity is anteromedialized. Usually no more than 1 cm of medialization is needed. Temporary stabilization is achieved with a Steinman pin placed lateral to the tibial tuberosity bone block. Fixation is achieved with two bicortical 4.5-mm cortical screws (Fig. 11.2).

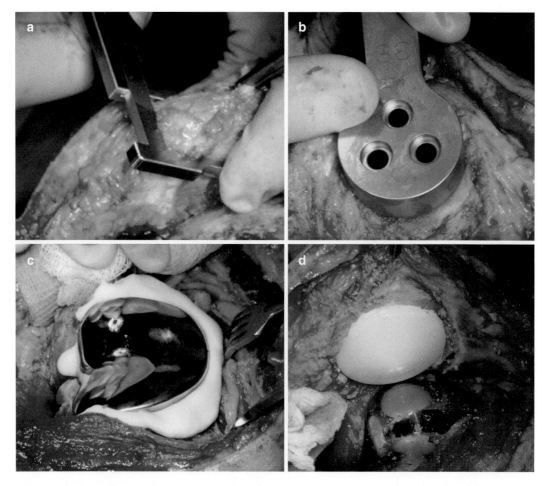

Fig. 11.4 Intraoperative pictures of the case described in Fig. 11.3. (**a**) Control of patellar resection and residual thickness. (**b**) Patellar sizing and preparation. (**c**) Definitive femoral component cementation. (**d**) Positioning of both components

11.2.5.2   Patellofemoral Arthroplasty (PFA)

If previous surgical scars do not need to be incorporated in the incision, a midline skin incision is performed to allow for future TKR. Quadriceps tendon, midvastus, and subvastus approaches may be used (Fig. 11.4). Some authors advocate the use of a lateral arthrotomy in order to better balance the lateral soft tissues after the implant. The patellar cut is performed first in order to allow for easier patellar dislocation during femoral preparation. All the osteophytes are removed, and the patellar cut is made to reestablish the original thickness with implant in place (Fig. 11.4a). For trochlear preparation, the first step is to remove the synovium, osteophytes, and fat from the anterior femur immediately adjacent to the most proximal extent of the trochlea. This allows direct visualization of the anterior femoral cortex, correct implant positioning, avoiding anterior femoral notching. If not markedly dysplastic, distal native trochlea is used for the femoral component orientation, together with the Whiteside's line and the transepicondylar axis. Some authors advocate 3° of external rotation as for the TKR, some others a neutral rotational alignment. If 3° external rotation is preferred, the "grand-piano" sign should be evident after the anterior femoral cut; on the contrary, if neutral rotation is planned, the cut femur typically presents the "butterfly sign." The trial components are then positioned, and tibial tubercle osteotomy is performed, if planned preoperatively. At this point, patellar tracking, possible tilt, and stability are checked throughout the complete range of motion of the knee. Soft tissue procedures (i.e., lateral release or medial reconstruction/plication) can be performed to treat these conditions. Possible clunking should be ruled out during the first 30° of flexion and at full flexion. The causes of the clunk may be (1) osteophytes, (2) soft tissues, and (3) femoral component malpositioning (undersizing or too superficial positioning of the inlay implant) [6]. Finally, definitive components can be implanted (Fig. 11.4).

11.2.5.3   Pearls and Pitfalls

Many of the patients undergoing surgery for PF pain had previous surgical procedures or trauma (fractures, dislocations, etc.), and attention should be paid to incorporate previous scars in the new incision and correctly balance the soft tissues, when performing a tibial tubercle osteotomy or a PFA.

Although there are no evidences about the amount of displacement required for the Fulkerson's osteotomy, overcorrection is not recommended, and an anteromedial displacement of 1–1.5 cm is usually sufficient to achieve good outcomes.

Correct component positioning, mainly on the femoral side, is mandatory in PFA: (1) excessive internal or external rotation should be avoided, and neutral or slight external (3°) rotation is the goal to achieve; (2) a correct sizing of the femoral component is important to avoid anterior femoral notching, (and 3) distal tip of the implant should not be prominent or below the roof of the notch.

When performing PFA, any malalignment, patellar tilt, or instability should be corrected concurrently, with the trial components positioned. After trial component placement, patellar tracking should be checked as well, applying a proximal traction to the quadriceps tendon [6].

11.2.6   Postoperative Regimen

Following a Fulkerson's osteotomy, immediate full weight bearing is protected by a hinged knee brace locked in full extension for 4–6 weeks. The brace can be removed 15 days after surgery to perform passive range of motion exercises.

Postoperative rehabilitation for PFA, lateral release, and facetectomy is straightforward, with early ROM exercises, muscle strengthening, and weight bearing as tolerated immediately after surgery.

11.2.7   Results

Total patellectomy showed to weaken the knee joint, require a long rehabilitation scheme for success, and compromise a following TKR. This surgical procedure can also leave residual pain, especially if trochlear changes are present. Although good to excellent results up to 87 % have been reported for patellectomy [4], this procedure should be avoided if possible in the young and active patient, because of the considerations mentioned above.

The excellent long-term results of TKR maintain debated the controversy between TKR and PFA in the treatment of isolated PF arthrosis in the older patient. However, newer PF implants and surgical techniques deliver good results beyond 10 years with failures predominantly resulting from tibiofemoral compartment arthritis progression [6]. Therefore, PFA is becoming an attractive and promising treatment option for isolated PF arthrosis in the young/active patient, without "burning bridges" for a subsequent TKR, if necessary. For the clinical results of specific implants, we refer to the recent review by Lustig [7].

11.2.8 Authors' Preferred Technique

The authors' indications for the treatment of isolated PF arthrosis are as follows:

- Conservative treatment: for all the patients, except in stage four arthrosis, where the beneficial effects of physical therapy are unpredictable.
- Arthroscopic debridement and lateral release: in patients with lateral tilt, PF lateral overload, and initial degenerative changes.
- Fulkerson's tibial tubercle osteotomy: in case of malalignment and arthrosis predominantly localized in the lateral PF joint. The osteotomy can be associated with (1) cartilage repair procedures (ACI, microfractures) in young patients (<40 years of age) with initial arthrosis or focal osteochondral defects and (2) PFA in older patients, if malalignment is present.
- Minimally invasive PFA: in patients with >40 years of age, central PF joint arthrosis, and no marked trochlear dysplasia.
- Traditional PFA: in patients with >40 years of age, diffuse PF joint arthrosis, and/or trochlear dysplasia.

11.3 Femorotibial Joint

11.3.1 Clinical Examination

History of the trauma, fracture, or knee surgery (arthroscopic debridement, meniscal or ligamentous surgery) needs to be clearly evaluated. Patients with femorotibial post-traumatic arthrosis typically report pain, swelling, catching, or locking, limited ROM as main symptoms. Initially, the pain is fluctuating and with mechanical features; increasing with weight bearing, walking, and sustained or sports activities; and decreasing with rest. Stiffness is common in the morning or when the patient starts walking after prolonged rest and usually improves after 30 min as well as with activity. As the degenerative process progresses, the periods of relief from symptoms become shorter, until the patients experience continuous and sometimes night pain.

On the physical examination, gait (showing limp or thrust), lower limb alignment, pain location, knee ROM, stability, and muscular strength should be evaluated. Malalignment, especially valgus, is common in the post-traumatic knee. Localized tenderness at the joint line and unicompartmental or widespread pain may be observed. To clinically assess the unicompartmental pain, the physician can use the "one-finger test" [8]. Patients can usually locate with one finger the tenderness point on the involved compartment. Otherwise, when the patient grabs the entire knee, often bicompartmental or tricompartmental arthrosis is present. Meniscal signs and stability tests need to be performed. Sometimes, unicompartmental knee arthrosis may mimic a meniscal injury in the involved compartment.

11.3.2 Imaging and Preoperative Workup

Radiographic evaluation includes bilateral weight-bearing anteroposterior (AP) views in full extension as well as tunnel views at 30° of flexion or Rosenberg views at 45° of flexion [9].

Lateral and skyline views are also obtained. A weight-bearing hip-to-ankle AP view is obtained to measure the lower extremity alignment. CT scan is usually required to better study the malunion and the intra-articular gap. MRI may be required to assess any other bony or soft tissue pathologies (meniscal tears, ligamentous lesions, osteochondral defects, avascular necrosis, etc.).

11.3.3 Classification

In 1980 Ahlbäck [10] popularized a widely used classification system for knee arthrosis, which includes five grades: (1) narrowing of the articular space, (2) obliteration or almost obliteration of the articular space, (3) bone attrition less than 5 mm, (4) bone attrition between 5 and 15 mm, and (5) bone attrition greater than 15 mm.

11.3.4 Indications

Whenever possible, reduction and resynthesis of inadequately reduced tibial plateau fractures should be performed (Fig. 11.5). However, in most cases articular damage is too advanced to perform such procedure, and surgeons have to deal with post-traumatic femorotibial arthrosis, following malunited fractures.

The treatments described for post-traumatic unicompartmental femorotibial arthrosis include (1) nonoperative management, (2) cartilage resurfacing procedure (Microfractures, OATS, ACI, and MACT), (3) high tibial osteotomy (HTO) and distal femoral osteotomy (DFO), (4) unicompartmental knee arthroplasty (UKA), and (5) unicondylar osteoarticular allografts.

11.3.4.1   Conservative Treatment
Conservative treatment is indicated in early stage of femorotibial arthrosis due to minimally displaced fractures, in slightly symptomatic patients or in older patients who feel they are doing well enough to avoid any surgical options. It is mainly focused on (1) weight loss, (2) physical therapy (quadriceps strengthening, muscles stretching, and maintenance of ROM), (3) analgesic and nonsteroidal anti-inflammatory drugs (NSAIDs), (4) unloading bracing (most of all if malalignment is present), and (5) intra-articular injections (corticosteroids and viscosupplementation).

11.3.4.2   Osteotomies
In the young patient (<40 years old) with early degenerative changes of the femorotibial compartment, cartilage resurfacing procedure can be performed alone or combined with HTO/DFO. In the treatment of unicompartmental knee arthrosis associated with malalignment, osteotomies

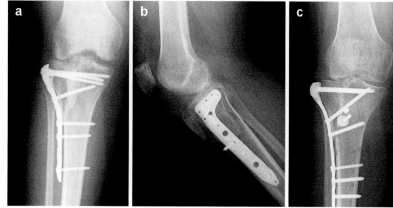

Fig. 11.5 Lateral tibial plateau malunion and tibial tuberosity nonunion. (**a, b**) Preoperative *AP* and lateral views; (**c, d**) postoperative *AP* and lateral views, after debridement, elevation of the lateral plateau, resynthesis of the tibial tuberosity and lateral plateau

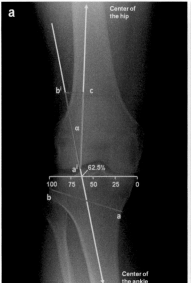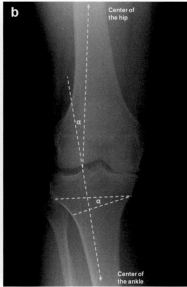

Fig. 11.6 Particular of weight-bearing long leg radiograph for the planning of HTO. (**a**) Planning for opening wedge HTO. The alignment should be corrected of an alpha angle, in order to obtain a weight-bearing line passing through the 62.5 % of the width of the tibial plateau. The osteotomy line (*ab*) is defined from medial (≈4 cm below the joint line) to lateral (tip of the fibular head). The line segment *ab* is transferred to the rays of the alpha angle from the vertex, in order to obtain the 2 line segments a^ib^i and a^ic. The distance b^ic is measured in millimeters and corresponds to the opening that should be achieved medially at the osteotomy site. (**b**) Planning for closing wedge HTO. The alpha angle is calculated and transferred to the osteotomy site on the proximal tibia, in order to have a triangle with lateral base

(HTO and DFO) are indicated for the patients with (1) age <60 years, (2) active lifestyle, (3) isolated mild lateral (or medial) knee arthritis (I or II in according with the Ahlback classification), (4) good ROM (knee flexion >120°), (5) no flexion contracture, and (6) intact medial (or lateral) and patellofemoral compartment. Many techniques have been described in the literature (opening wedge, closing wedge, dome, and progressive callus distraction with external fixator). In the treatment of the varus knee, opening wedge high tibial osteotomy (OWHTO) and closing wedge high tibial osteotomy (CWHTO) are the most commonly used techniques for corrections of malalignment up to 15°. In the treatment of lateral compartment arthrosis and valgus malalignment of the knee, lateral opening wedge distal femoral osteotomy (OWDFO) and medial closing wedge distal femoral medial osteotomy (CWDFO) have been described. When larger valgus or varus correction (>15°) is needed, dome osteotomy or progressive callus distraction with monoaxial or Taylor frame external fixator is indicated. The preoperative planning for osteotomies around the knee is described in Figs. 11.6 and 11.7.

11.3.5 Surgical Techniques

11.3.5.1 Surgical Technique for Medial OWHTO

Concurrent arthroscopy can be performed to evaluate and treat any intra-articular pathologies (Figs. 11.8 and 11.9). A 5–8 cm longitudinal skin incision is made from 1 cm below the medial joint line midway between the medial border of the tubercle and the posteromedial aspect of the tibia (Fig. 11.9). The sartorial fascia is incised, and the anterior portion of the superficial medial collateral ligament is elevated. The patellar tendon is protected throughout the whole procedure. A guide wire is placed across the proximal tibia from medial

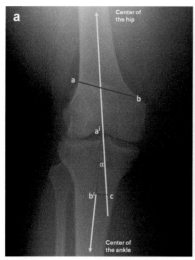 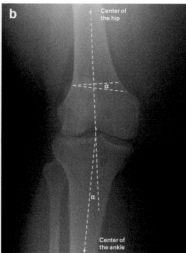

Fig. 11.7 Particular of weight-bearing long leg radiograph for the planning of DFO. (**a**) Planning for lateral opening wedge DFO. The alignment should be corrected of an alpha angle, in order to obtain a weight-bearing line passing in the middle of the joint. The osteotomy line (*ab*) is defined, and the line segment *ab* is transferred to the rays of the alpha angle from the vertex, in order to obtain the two line segments $a^i b^i$ and $a^i c$. The distance $b^i c$ is measured in millimeters and corresponds to the opening that should be achieved laterally at the osteotomy site. (**b**) Planning for medial closing wedge DFO. The alpha angle is calculated and transferred to the osteotomy site on distal femur, in order to have a triangle with medial base

to lateral under fluoroscopic control (Fig. 11.9). The wire is positioned on the superior aspect of the tibial tubercle and oriented obliquely to 1 cm below the joint line at the lateral tibial cortex. The anterior and medial cortices are cut with an oscillating saw below the wire (Fig. 11.9). The direction of osteotomy should be parallel to the tibial slope. The osteotomy is deepened with osteotomes under fluoroscopic control and the medial opening is obtained using a special wedge-shaped spreader (Fig. 11.9). An intact lateral hinge is required to improve the stability of the osteotomy. Intraoperative alignment is checked intermittently under fluoroscopy and, once the desired correction is achieved, with an alignment rod centered on the hip and ankle joints. At the level of the knee, the rod should pass over the lateral tibial spine, as preoperatively planned. The osteotomy can be fixed with locked or butterfly plates, with or without spacers (Figs. 11.8 and 11.9). The osseous gap can be filled with allograft, autograft, or synthetic bone substitutes in case of large opening.

11.3.5.2 Surgical Technique for Lateral CWHTO

An anterolateral L-shaped incision is performed with the vertical part along the lateral edge of the tibial tubercle and the horizontal one parallel to the lateral joint line (1 cm distal). The fascia of the anterolateral compartment is incised; the tibialis anterior muscle and the iliotibial band are elevated proximally. The common peroneal nerve and the patellar tendon are protected throughout the procedure. Many techniques have been described for the proximal tibiofibular joint, including (1) joint excision or disruption, (2) fibular osteotomy (10 cm distal from the fibular head), and (3) excision of the fibular head. Then, a laterally based wedge can be removed with an angular cutting guide. In order to reduce the risk of intra-articular fracture, the outer cortex and large portion of the wedge can be removed with saw cuts, along with the medial half using a combination of curettes, rongeurs, and osteotomes, to within 1 cm of the medial cortex. The completeness of wedge removal must be assessed fluoroscopically. The closure of the osteotomy can be performed and the alignment checked with the fluoroscope. Fixation is then achieved with staples or a plate [11].

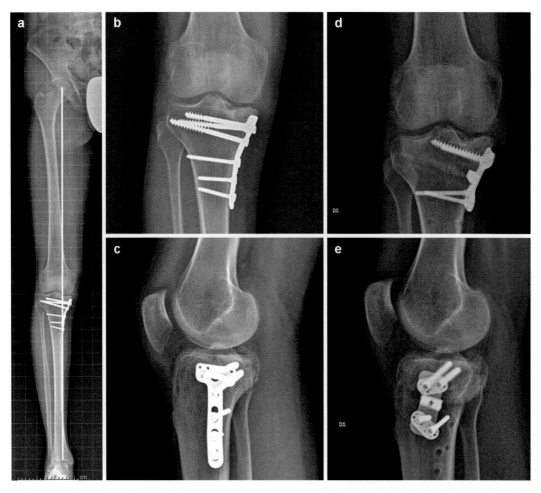

Fig. 11.8 Medial tibial plateau malunion. (**a**) Long leg AP X-ray view showing varus malalignment; (**b, c**) preoperative AP and lateral views; (**d, e**) postoperative *AP* and lateral views, after opening wedge HTO

11.3.5.3 Surgical Technique for Lateral OWDFO

A 10–15 cm longitudinal lateral distal femoral incision is performed starting 2 cm distal to the femoral condyle and prolonging it proximally. The iliotibial band is split to the level of the joint line, and the vastus lateralis is retracted from the intermuscular septum using a curve blunt retractor placed ventrally. The bone plane is better exposed with a slight knee flexion. Under fluoroscopic control (Fig. 11.10), a guide wire is inserted in the middle of the lateral femur, with a cranio-caudal inclination of 20°, from lateral (6–7 cm above the joint line) to medial (4–5 cm above the joint line). The exposed cortex is cut with a small oscillating saw above the guide wire

(Fig. 11.10). Sharp and thin AO osteotomes are then used to complete the osteotomy to within 1 cm from the medial cortex, under fluoroscopic guidance. The site of osteotomy at this point is opened with a wedge opener to the desired correction. Fluoroscopy and alignment rod are used to assess the limb correction, as previously described. A distal femoral osteotomy plate (regular or locked) is then used for fixation (Fig. 11.10). Bone grafting or bone substitutes are used to fill the gap [12].

11.3.5.4 Surgical Technique for Medial CWDFO

A longitudinal 10–15 cm anteromedial incision is performed on the distal femur. The fascia over

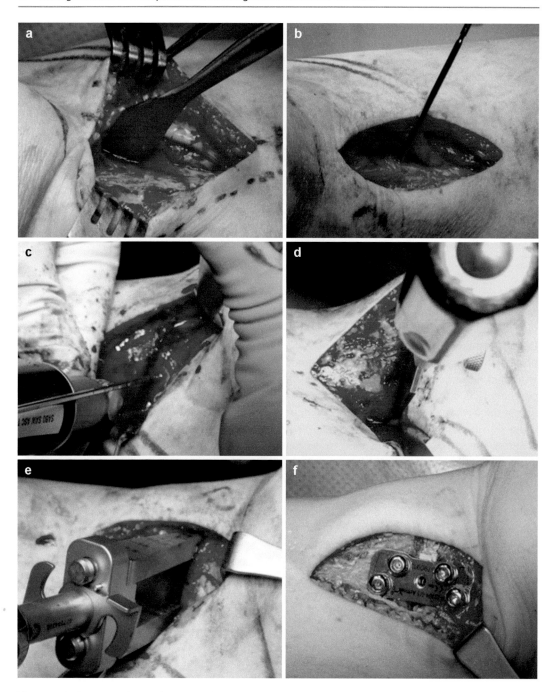

Fig. 11.9 Intraoperative pictures of OWHTO. (**a**) Elevation of the sartorial fascia, hamstrings, and anterior part of the sMCL. (**b**) Guide wire positioning under fluoroscopic control. (**c**) Antero- and posteromedial cortex cut with oscillating saw, below the K wire and protecting the patellar tendon with a Hohmann retractor. (**d**) Completion of the HTO with graduated chisels. (**e**) Graduated wedge-shaped osteotomy spreader inserted to open the osteotomy site. (**f**) Fixation of the osteotomy with butterfly plate and augmentation with bone substitutes

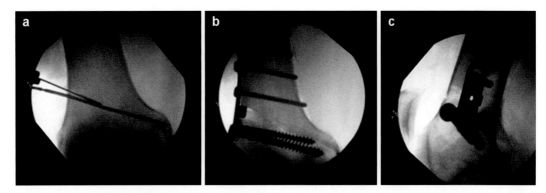

Fig. 11.10 Surgical technique for lateral OWDFO. (**a**) Guide wire insertion under fluoroscopic control. Cut of the cortex with a small oscillating saw above the guide wire. (**b, c**) The site of osteotomy is opened with a wedge opener, and fixation is achieved with a toothed plate. Final anteroposterior (**b**) and lateral (**c**) control, after allograft bone augmentation

the vastus medialis muscle is incised, and the muscle is separated from the intermuscular septum and retracted superiorly. A guide wire is inserted parallel to the joint line. A slot for a blade plate is then prepared parallel to the guide wire, and an osteotomy is made about 2–3 cm proximal to it. The medial cortex and large portion of the wedge can be removed with saw cuts, along with the medial half using a combination of curettes, rongeurs, and osteotomes, to within 1 cm of the medial cortex. A 90° angle blade plate is inserted in the prepared slot. Manual varus reduction is performed, allowing the medial spike of the proximal part to dig into the distal cancellous bone. The rigid fixation is achieved with the anatomic knee axis of 0°, after fluoroscopic assessment of the correction.

11.3.5.5 Surgical Technique for Large Corrections (Progressive Callus Distraction or Dome Osteotomy)

When larger correction (>15°) is required, either a progressive callus distraction or a dome osteotomy can be performed. In the progressive callus distraction, the fixation can be achieved with a monoaxial external fixator or with a Taylor frame hybrid ring fixator, with the latter allowing for a more stable construct and a better correction on the three planes. Bolsters are placed under the thigh and foot, allowing for circumferential access to the tibia from the knee to the ankle. The frame is sized and constructed preoperatively and is checked once more to ensure appropriate fit on the patient's leg. A fine wire is passed from lateral to medial parallel to the joint surface, at least 10 mm distal to the joint. The frame is applied to this wire and, using the undersurface of the frame as a template, a second fine wire is passed, taking care to keep the frame parallel to the joint surface in coronal and sagittal planes. The frame is then secured distally using a fine wire across the distal ring. The construct is then completed by adding two 5-mm half pins to each ring. The osteotomy is then performed percutaneously at the lower border of the tibial tubercle, through two small incisions using a Gigli saw subperiosteally. The osteotomy is left static for 10 days after which the correction is then performed gradually by the patient at home, usually over a 7–14-day period, depending on the degree of deformity. The frame is removed after healing is confirmed radiologically and clinically [13]. In the dome osteotomy, a 7–8 cm midline skin incision is made from the level of the joint line to 3 cm below the tibial tubercle. The anterior tibia is exposed medial and lateral to the patellar tendon, which is protected throughout the whole procedure. The inverse U-shaped osteotomy site is marked with the cautery, with the apex above the tibial tubercle. Multiple holes are drilled with a 2-mm drill from anterior to posterior along the osteotomy line, to weaken the anterior and posterior cortices. A small osteotome is used to complete the

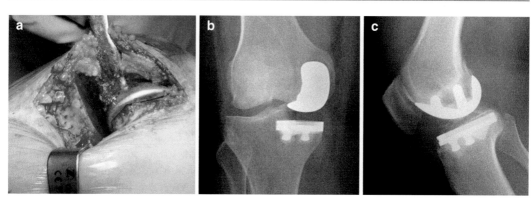

Fig. 11.11 Severe medial compartment arthrosis of the knee. (**a**) Intraoperative picture, during UKA implant. (**b, c**) Postoperative anteroposterior and lateral views after UKA implant

osteotomy anteriorly and posteriorly. The correction maneuver is performed and the alignment controlled with an alignment rod fluoroscopically. Occasionally, the proximal tibiofibular joint needs to be disrupted in order to obtain the desired correction. Alternatively, a fibular osteotomy may be done 10 cm distal to the fibular head through an additional lateral incision. The osteotomy can be fixed with a plate or an external fixator. In the latter case, the proximal pins should be positioned parallel to the joint line, before performing the osteotomy.

11.3.5.6 Unicompartmental Knee Arthroplasty (UKA)

Even though osteotomy and UKA are sometimes considered alternative treatment options for the treatment of unicompartmental knee arthrosis, the indications in most of the cases are different, and only a small population of patients is amenable to both treatments. Ideal indications for UKA include (1) unicompartmental arthrosis (no matter which stage), with both lateral and patellofemoral compartments intact; (2) age >60 years; (3) low demands; (4) no overweight; (5) minimal pain at rest; (6) ROM >90°; (7) less than 5° flexion contracture; (8) less than 10° of axial malalignment that can however be passively corrected to almost neutral; and (9) no instability. A 6–10 cm medial parapatellar skin incision is performed, extending from the superior pole of the patella to about 2–4 cm below the joint line adjacent to the tibial tubercle (Fig. 11.11). A subvastus

approach to the joint is commonly used. Even though some authors suggest an anterolateral approach for lateral compartment UKA, a slightly more extensile medial parapatellar approach allows for lateral compartment exposure. The patella is then dislocated, possibly without eversion, and all the osteophytes removed. The anterior horn of the meniscus and the fat pad are removed to optimize visualization. At this point, many techniques have been described for distal femoral and proximal tibial cuts preparation. Although most commonly the tibial cut is performed first, a femur-first bone preparation can be performed with an intramedullary or extramedullary technique. When a tibia-first bone preparation technique is preferred, the tibial cut is performed perpendicular to the tibial shaft with an ankle clamp extramedullary tibial guide. A 5° tibial slope is usually maintained, although reducing the tibial slope may help to achieve a complete ROM in patients with flexion contracture. After the tibial preparation, a dependent femoral cut can be performed with a spacer block, positioned parallel to the tibial cut, or with an extramedullary technique, adding the femoral resector to the extramedullary guide previously used. An independent femoral cut can be performed with an intramedullary technique. Flexion and extension gaps should be checked out with spacers, to assess the need for recut or soft tissue balancing. After a correct sizing, the femoral preparation is completed, the trial components are positioned, and ROM together with limb alignment is controlled. Final components are then cemented. Either metal backed or all poly tibial components are available, according to the implant selected.

11.3.5.7 Unicondylar Osteoarticular Allografts and Osteotomy

In case of young patients (<40 years of age) with large post-traumatic tibial or femoral articular defects, unicondylar osteoarticular allografts can be indicated (Figs. 11.12, 11.13, 11.14, and 11.15). The opposite articular surface needs to be preserved, when performing unicondylar grafting. The X-rays and CT scan of the patient are sent to the tissue bank for correct sizing of the fresh allograft. Exposure of the recipient knee is performed through a midline skin incision followed by a parapatellar arthrotomy to expose the affected tibial or femoral condyle. The damaged condyle is resected to bleeding bone, while the donor fragment is trimmed to fit the defect. The graft is usually fixed with partially threaded 3.5-mm cancellous screws. During tibial plateau transplantation, the meniscus is evaluated and, when severely damaged, replaced with the allograft meniscus attached to the donor plateau. Already attached to its own osseous anchors, the meniscus is repaired to the capsule with the use of absorbable sutures. Realignment of the involved lower limb needs to be performed to unload the graft, if standing radiographs show a weight-bearing line passing through the involved compartment (Figs. 11.12 and 11.13). A valgus or varus closing wedge osteotomy is performed in the bone opposite to the defect (i.e., femoral osteotomy for tibial plateau osteoarticular allografts) [14, 15].

11.3.6 Postoperative Regimen

In HTO and DFO, active range of motion in a hinged knee brace and toe-touch weight bearing are allowed immediately. Partial weight bearing with crutches or total weight bearing as tolerated is allowed at 6 weeks, according to radiographic evidence of bone healing, amount of opening, and stability of the osteotomy (preserved medial or lateral hinges, use of locking plates). With progressive callus distraction technique, range of motion as tolerated is allowed immediately, and weight bearing is restricted for the first 10 days, while pin tracts heal. Thereafter, partial weight bearing with crutches is allowed. At the end of the initial correction, a long-standing weight-bearing film is taken, parameters are entered into the computer software, and any necessary residual correction can be done until optimal alignment is achieved. The frame is removed after healing is confirmed radiographically and clinically.

In UKA weight bearing, ROM exercises and muscle strengthening are immediately allowed and progressed as tolerated. Postoperative regimen for unicondylar osteoarticular allografts includes a 2-week period of cylinder cast immobilization, followed by ROM exercises in an unlocked hinged knee brace. Partial weight bearing is allowed in the brace after union of the osteotomy site, usually at 3 months after surgery.

11.3.7 Results

Controversy still exists regarding which technique has to be preferred between CWHTO and OWHTO, for the treatment of medial knee arthrosis and varus malalignment. Lateral CWHTO has been considered for a long time as the gold standard. However, this technique implies (1) fibular osteotomy or proximal tibiofibular joint disruption, (2) lateral muscle detachment, (3) peroneal nerve dissection, (4) more demanding subsequent total joint replacement, and (5) bone stock loss. For all these reasons, the medial OWHTO gained popularity and became a widely used alternative option. This technique however is not free from drawbacks, and these include the necessity of bone graft and possible collapse or loss of correction [16]. Further advantages of OWHTO include the possibility for multiplanar correction and treatment of combined ligamentous instability. However, no conclusion can be drawn on which technique is to be preferred, and the choice remains a matter of preference of the surgeon,

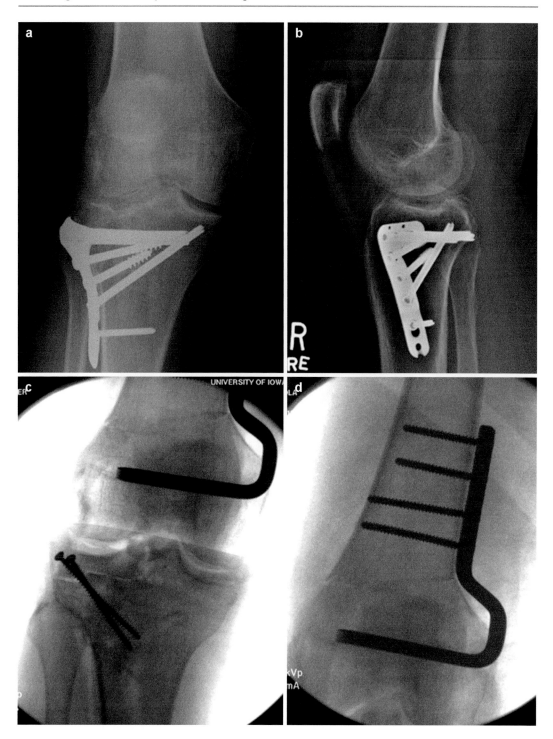

Fig. 11.12 Severe post-traumatic lateral tibial plateau degeneration and valgus malalignment. (**a, b**) Preoperative anteroposterior and lateral views, showing malunion with valgus malalignment. (**c, d**) Intraoperative image intensifier views after unicondylar lateral tibial plateau allograft and medial CWDFO

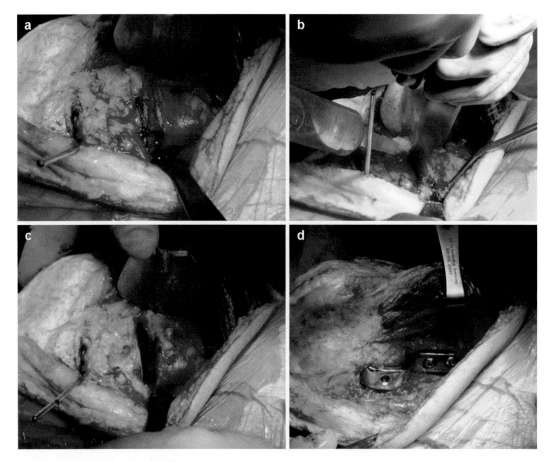

Fig. 11.13 Intraoperative pictures of the case described in Fig. 11.12 (CWDFO phase). (**a**) A guide wire is inserted parallel to the joint line, and the slot for the blade plate is then prepared parallel to the guide wire. (**b, c**) The oste-otomy is made about 2–3 cm proximal to the wire. (**d**) A 90° angle blade plate is inserted in the prepared slot, and manual varus reduction is performed

until further studies become available in the literature.

Other controversies regarding unicompartmental knee arthrosis include the graft selection and type of fixation in OWHTO, the comparison between UKA and osteotomy, and whether HTO or UKA affects a subsequent total joint replacement, which represents the endpoint for both failed treatments.

Both osteotomy and UKA showed satisfactory results and survival rates at mid- and long-term follow-up. A few papers attempted to make a comparison between the two procedures and generally showed slightly better results for UKA, in terms of survivorship and functional outcome. Nevertheless, the differences are not remarkable,

and the quality of these studies is insufficient to draw any definitive conclusion. Furthermore, we believe that UKA and osteotomy are different procedures with different indications, and a comparison between them is meaningful only in the small population of patients amenable to both treatments. This population includes patients who are (1) from 60 to 65 years old, (2) moderately active, and (3) nonobese and (4) with mild varus malalignment (from 5 to 10°), (5) without joint instability, (6) with a good range of motion, and (7) with moderate unicompartmental arthritis [17, 18].

Whether revision HTO or UKA to TKA performs worse than primary TKA is a debated issue. Given that TKA represents the endpoint of every failed HTO or UKA, this aspect is particularly

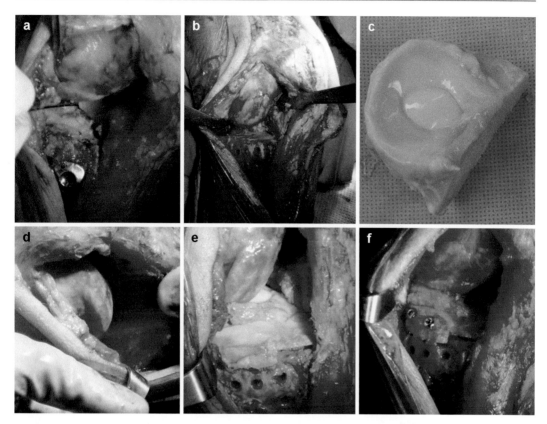

Fig. 11.14 Intraoperative pictures of the case described in Figs. 11.12 and, 11.13 (unicondylar tibial plateau allograft phase). (**a**) Note the large defect in the lateral tibial plateau and the plate previously used to fix the lateral tibial plateau fracture. (**b**) Resection of the damaged lateral plateau and hardware removal. (**c**) Fresh frozen tibial plateau allograft with the lateral meniscus attached. (**d**) Preparation of a step in the tibial bone cut, in order to improve the allograft stability. (**e**) Insertion of the graft in the joint. (**f**) Fixation with 2 screws

important. Both revision HTO and revision UKA to TKA are technically more challenging than primary TKA: (1) HTO in terms of surgical exposure and tibial component positioning and (2) UKA in terms of bone stock loss and need for bone grafting both on the femoral and the tibial side. While HTO does not seem to affect the results of subsequent TKA, revision UKA to TKA apparently performs worse than primary TKA. It has to be mentioned here that all the studies in the English literature reported the results of TKA after CWHTO and no data are available about TKA after OWHTO. This is an important issue because, theoretically, TKA is easier after opening wedge HTO than after closing wedge HTO. Indeed, with opening wedge HTO, there is no risk of patella alta, the bone stock is maintained, and the risk of impingement between the tibial stem and the anterior tibial cortex is decreased [17].

The results of unicondylar osteoarticular allografts and osteotomy were recently described by Drexler et al. [15–19].

Fig. 11.15 Lateral tibial plateau malunion with valgus malalignment. (**a**) Long leg AP X-ray view showing valgus malalignment; (**b**) preoperative coronal CT scan; (**c**) postoperative AP view, after lateral opening DFO and fresh frozen tibial plateau (with the lateral meniscus) allograft transplant

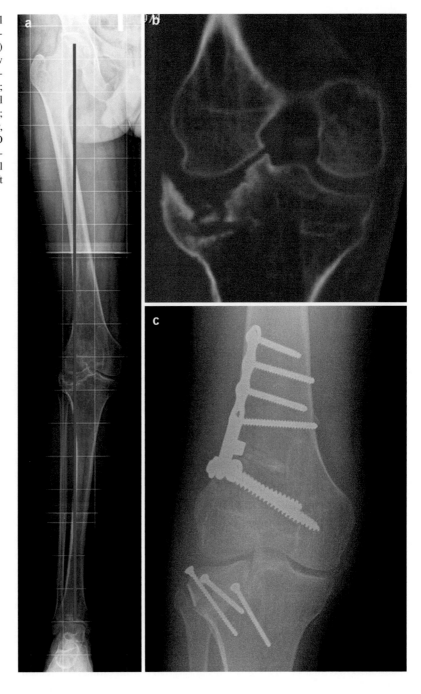

References

1. Aglietti P, Insall JN, Cerulli G (1983) Patellar pain and incongruence. I: measurements of incongruence. Clin Orthop Relat Res 176:217–224
2. Dejour D, Le Coltre B (2007) Osteotomies in patellofemoral instabilities. Sports Med Arthrosc 15:39–46
3. Merchant AC, Mercer RL, Jacobsen RG, Cool CR (1974) Roentgenographic analysis of patellofemoral congruence. J Bone Joint Surg Am 56: 1391–1396
4. Donell ST, Glasgow MM (2007) Isolated patellofemoral osteoarthritis. Knee 14:169–176
5. Cannon A, Stolley M, Wolf B, Amendola A (2008) Patellofemoral resurfacing arthroplasty: literature

review and description of a novel technique. Iowa Orthop J 28:42–48

6. Farr J 2nd, Barrett D (2008) Optimizing patellofemoral arthroplasty. Knee 15:339–347

7. Lustig S (2014) Patellofemoral arthroplasty. Orthop Traumatol Surg Res 100(1 Suppl):S35–S43

8. Bert JM (2005) Unicompartmental knee replacement. Orthop Clin North Am 36:513–522

9. Rosenberg TD, Paulos LE, Parker RD et al (1988) The forty-five degree posteroanterior flexion weight-bearing radiograph of the knee. J Bone Joint Surg Am 70:1479–1483

10. Ahlbäck S, Rydberg J (1980) Röntgenologisk klassifikation och undersökningsteknik vid gonartros. Lakartidningen 77:2091–2096

11. Rossi R, Bonasia DE, Amendola A (2011) The role of high tibial osteotomy in the varus knee. J Am Acad Orthop Surg 19:590–599

12. Phisitkul P, Wolf BR, Amendola A (2006) Role of high tibial and distal femoral osteotomies in the treatment of lateral-posterolateral and medial instabilities of the knee. Sports Med Arthrosc 14:96–104

13. Amendola A (2003) The role of osteotomy in the multiple ligament injured knee. Arthroscopy 19 Supp l:11–13

14. Shasha N, Krywulak S, Backstein D, Pressman A, Gross AE (2003) Long-term follow-up of fresh tibial osteochondral allografts for failed tibial plateau fractures. J Bone Joint Surg Am 85:33–39

15. Drexler M, Gross A, Dwyer T, Safir O, Backstein D, Chaudhry H, Goulding A, Kosashvili Y (2015) Distal femoral varus osteotomy combined with tibial plateau fresh osteochondral allograft for post-traumatic osteoarthritis of the knee. Knee Surg Sports Traumatol Arthrosc 23:1317–23

16. Amendola A, Bonasia DE (2010) Results of high tibial osteotomy: review of the literature. Int Orthop 34:155–160

17. Dettoni F, Bonasia DE, Castoldi F, Bruzzone M, Blonna D, Rossi R (2010) High tibial osteotomy versus unicompartmental knee arthroplasty for medial compartment arthrosis of the knee: a review of the literature. Iowa Orthop J 30:131–140

18. Lustig S, Parratte S, Magnussen RA, Argenson JN, Neyret P (2012) Lateral unicompartmental knee arthroplasty relieves pain and improves function in posttraumatic osteoarthritis. Clin Orthop Relat Res 470(1):69–76

19. Raz G, Safir OA, Backstein DJ, Lee PT, Gross AE (2014) Distal femoral fresh osteochondral allografts: follow-up at a mean of twenty-two years. J Bone Joint Surg Am 96(13):1101–1107

Management of the Complications Following Fractures Around the Knee (Post-traumatic Bi- or Tricompartmental Arthritis)

12

Federica Rosso, Umberto Cottino, Matteo Bruzzone, Federico Dettoni, and Roberto Rossi

Abstract

The relationship between periarticular fractures and development of knee arthritis is well known. However, considering the lack of the literature, it is difficult to precisely estimate the incidence of post-traumatic arthritis of the knee, ranging from 20 % at 5 years to 50 % at 15 years after the fracture. A treatment option for most of the patients could be total knee arthroplasty (TKA). In these patients, the strategy should be accurately planned preoperatively, because of different problems: presence of hardware, multiple surgical scars, bony defects, malalignment, stiffness, instability, malunions, previous infections, and ligamentous deficiency. TKA after proximal tibial or distal femoral fractures can be challenging, most of all for bone loss and instability. The results of post-traumatic TKA are good, but more similar to revision TKA than to standard primary TKA. Post-traumatic TKA patients have a higher risk of complications compared to the general population undergoing TKA for primary osteoarthritis. It is still unclear whether post-traumatic TKAs have a higher risk of infection compared to standard TKAs, but a higher risk of infection in TKAs after infected periarticular fractures has been reported.

Keywords

Knee arthroplasty • Post-traumatic arthritis • Complex knee • Complication

F. Rosso (✉) • M. Bruzzone • F. Dettoni
AO Mauriziano Umberto I,
SCDU Ortopedia e Traumatologia,
Largo Turati 62, Torino 10128, Italy
e-mail: federica.rosso@yahoo.it

U. Cottino
Dipartimento di Scienze Chirurgiche,
Università degli Studi di Torino,
Via Po 8, Torino 10100, Italy

R. Rossi
AO Mauriziano Umberto I,
SCDU Ortopedia e Traumatologia,
Largo Turati 62, Torino 10128, Italy

Dipartimento di Scienze Chirurgiche,
Università degli Studi di Torino,
Via Po 8, Torino 10100, Italy

© Springer International Publishing Switzerland 2016
F. Castoldi, D.E. Bonasia (eds.), *Fractures Around the Knee*, Fracture Management Joint by Joint,
DOI 10.1007/978-3-319-28806-2_12

12.1   Epidemiology

Different authors reported that articular incongruity and instability can lead to post-traumatic arthritis [7, 16, 31].

There are few long-term studies on arthritis after proximal tibial or distal femoral fractures, and the incidence is not clearly defined. Honkonen et al. in 1995 reported an incidence of 44 % for post-traumatic arthritis in 131 cases, at 7.6 years after surgically treated fractures around the knee. The authors reported young age, combined meniscectomy, medial tilt, articular cartilage damage, inadequate fixation, residual malalignment, and poor reduction as risk factors for developing post-traumatic osteoarthritis [7, 14]. Conversely, Wasserstein et al. observed a 5.3 times increased risk of total knee arthroplasty (TKA) in patients affected by a proximal tibial plateau fracture 10 years before compared to standard population, with a further increased risk correlated to old age (hazard risk, HR, 1.03 per year over the age of 48), bicondylar fracture (HR 1.53), and major comorbidities (HR 2.17) [45]. Other authors reported an incidence of arthritis ranging between 20 % at 5 years and 50 % at 15 years after a proximal tibial fracture [21, 34]. A similar incidence of post-traumatic arthritis was estimated after treatment of comminuted, intra-articular fractures of the distal femur [30, 39].

However, different authors reported that the development of end-stage knee post-traumatic osteoarthritis occurs at a mean of 7 years after the fracture, ranging from 2 to 11 years [20, 21] (Fig. 12.1).

12.2   Clinical Examination

When approaching a TKA in a patient with previous surgery, the strategy should take into account different problems: the presence of hardware, multiple surgical scars, bony defects, malalignment, stiffness, instability, malunions, and previous infections [3]. For these reasons, delayed TKA in patients with previous periarticular knee fractures can be challenging, with a 26 % rate of complication and 21 % of reoperation [47].

Clinical examination should include the evaluation of location and type of pain, degree and type of instability, gait disturbance, or malalignment. Preoperative range of motion (ROM) evaluation is mandatory: post-traumatic arthritis can be associated with limitation of flexion or extension [27, 28]. The patients should be informed on the realistic expectation for postoperative ROM because this is correlated with the preoperative movement [17]. Previous scars, the need for a skin graft, or other cutaneous problems should be carefully evaluated, because of the higher risk of cutaneous complication in these patients. In case of complex previous surgeries, with multiple skin incision, the plastic surgeon should be consulted [3].

Furthermore, post-traumatic arthritis can be associated with extensor mechanism abnormalities, i.e., patella baja, due to fibrous tissue formation and consequent stiffness [3] (Fig. 12.2).

12.3   Imaging and Preoperative Workup

The first step is to obtain a complete radiographic study including anteroposterior (AP), lateral, Merchant, and long-leg weight-bearing views. On the x-rays, the surgeon should evaluate bone stock, patellar height, osteolysis, hardware position, limb alignment, and significant bony deformities below or above the joint [35]. Some authors described the tilt of the tibial plateau in the AP and lateral views as an important aspect, reporting patients with a medial tilt having a higher risk of developing post-traumatic arthritis [14]. In our experience, a computed tomography (CT) scan is fundamental to evaluate bone quality, bony defects, and hardware position. In patients with a history of open fracture or previous septic joint, considering the high suspicion of infection, a blood count with differential, erythrocyte sedimentation rate (ESR), C-reactive protein level (CRP), and joint aspiration should be performed to rule out active infections [3, 4].

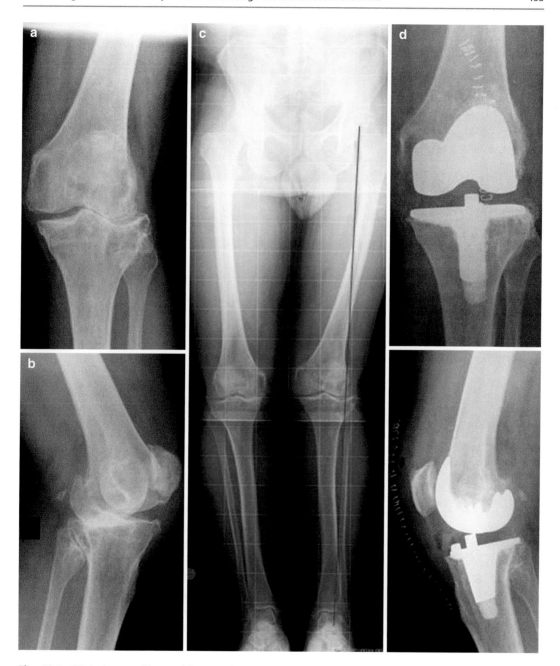

Fig. 12.1 Clinical case: 54-year-old man with post-traumatic left knee arthritis after previous lateral plateau fracture. (**a**) Preoperative anteroposterior (AP) x-ray; (**b**) lateral preoperative view; (**c**) preoperative long-leg view showing the valgus malalignment; (**d**) postoperative x-rays

12.4   Indications

Proximal tibial plateau fractures are common in patients younger than 50 years old [9]. Consequently a considerable number of patients affected by post-traumatic arthritis can be younger than 60 years, and this complicates the treatment choice. In patients younger than 60 years, with uni-compartimental post-traumatic arthritis, osteotomies around the knee may

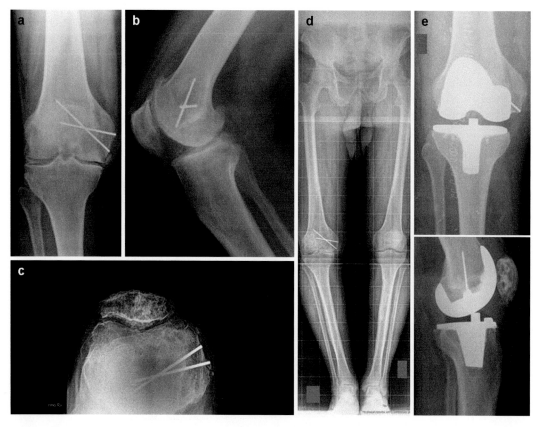

Fig. 12.2 Clinical case: 75-year-old man with post-traumatic right knee arthritis after previous distal femoral and patellar fracture. (**a**) Preoperative anteroposterior (AP) x-ray showing the retained hardware; (**b**) lateral preoperative view showing a patella baja; (**c**) preoperative patellar view; (**d**) preoperative long-leg view; (**e**) postoperative x-rays

decrease pain and slow down the progression to arthritis, delaying the time for a total knee arthroplasty [1, 12].

However, in all patients affected by bi- or tricompartmental post-traumatic arthritis, a TKA should be considered. There is still a debate on the best approach for hardware removal, which is often necessary because of its interference with the implant or the instrumentation. When extensive hardware removal is required, especially in cases with poor skin quality, a two-step surgery is recommended: first step of hardware removal, followed by TKA after soft tissue recovery. The same approach should be considered in the cases with suspected infection [3, 48].

12.5   Implant Selection

Similarly to primary TKA, different joint arthroplasty designs can be considered in post-traumatic bi- or tricompartmental arthritis. The implant with the least constraint necessary to provide symmetric, well-balanced flexion and extension gaps should be preferred [3].

Posterior cruciate ligament (PCL) retaining (cruciate retaining, CR) implants can be used in selected cases with minimal deformities, no flexion contractures, and no instabilities. However, in the vast majority of the cases, a posterior-stabilized (PS) implant allows for deformity correction and accurate ligament balancing [3, 7]. In patients affected by arthrofibrosis or flexion deformity, a PS implant should be preferred [4].

When ligamentous deficiencies or poor bone quality is present, a more constrained implant may be required in association with femoral or tibial extensions. In cases with poor bone quality, but good ligamentous balance, a standard PS design can be used, in association with stem extensions and bone fillers, e.g., wedges and sleeves [4]. Hinged implants should be reserved to patients with low activity level, severe instability, or major bone loss [40].

12.6   Surgical Technique

When performing a TKA after a tibial plateau fracture, different problems should be considered: prior incisions, hardware removal, alignment, instability, and bony defects. In this section, the differences between TKA in post-traumatic arthritis and standard TKA will be discussed.

12.6.1   Prior Incisions

The presence of prior incisions should be carefully evaluated in the preoperative planning. Considering the vascular supply of the anterior knee skin, the most recent or most lateral incision should be chosen, avoiding the elevation of large subcutaneous flaps [3, 15, 29]. Old transverse skin scars should not be transected creating acute angle ≤60° because triangular skin flaps have a high risk of necrosis. When a new incision is required, the surgeon should create a skin bridge of at least 6 cm [3, 15].

12.6.2   Exposure

Post-traumatic arthritis can be associated with a stiff knee. In these cases, the general principles for stiff knee exposure should be followed, including the following: (1) protection of patellar tendon; (2) sequential release of scarring in the suprapatellar space, gutters, and peritendinous

tissue; and (3) avoiding vigorous retraction or forceful flexion of the knee [3]. The so-called Tarabichi maneuver can be useful to remove the adhesions of the quadriceps muscle [43]. When the quadriceps is severely contracted, a V-Y turndown or tibial tubercle osteotomy can be highly effective to gain adequate exposure. If a V-Y quadriceps turndown is chosen, the surgeon should pay attention to the superior lateral geniculate artery, to reduce the risk of devascularization of the patellar and patellar tendon. On the other hand, when performing a tibial tubercle osteotomy, the fragment should be approximately 2 cm wide and 8–10 mm thick, and care should be taken to preserve the lateral soft tissue hinge [10, 27].

12.6.3 Malalignment

Intra-articular deformity correction should follow the general principles of TKA. It is mandatory to obtain a well-aligned lower limb: many authors demonstrated an increased risk of mechanical failure and aseptic loosening when components or mechanical axis shows malalignment postoperatively [21].

Conversely, large deformities may require an extra-articular correction through an osteotomy, which can be performed in a staged or simultaneous procedure [23]. Rotational deformity is not rare in post-traumatic arthritis, and it should be carefully evaluated and corrected before or at the time of surgery [41]. Malalignment due to ligament incongruence can be managed as well as in revision TKA or in valgus-varus TKA. In these cases, a constrained implant may be required [4].

12.6.4 TKA in Nonunion

There is little data in literature regarding TKA after proximal tibial fracture nonunion. Some authors suggested to bypass the nonunion with longer stem in association with bone grafts. Small fragments can be excised, and the bone defect can be treated following the revision TKA principles [2, 18, 22, 50].

In some cases, intramedullary guides can be difficult to use, so extramedullary, navigation, or personalized instrumentations can be useful. Tumor prostheses can be used in elderly patients with large defects, nonunion, and bone fragments [25].

12.6.5 Bone Loss

Bone losses are frequent in post-traumatic arthritis and should be managed according to the principles of revision surgery [3]. Furthermore, metaphyseal bone is often compromised in post-traumatic arthritis, so the bone ingrowth in the cementless implants may be inadequate, and longer stems can be useful [21].

Contained small defects, less than 5 mm, can be filled with cement, while bigger defects can be managed using metallic augments, bone grafts, or tantalum cones [13, 33] (Fig. 12.3). Large cavitary metaphyseal deficiencies can be managed with tantalum cones, sleeves, or impaction graft techniques [3]. Many authors prefer metallic augments over bone allograft because of the better primary stability, earlier mobilization, and immediate weight bearing. Bone losses can also affect the joint line, causing impairment of the extensor mechanism function and gap imbalance of the implant. In these cases, metal augments can be very useful in restoring the correct joint line,

using the landmarks as described in revision TKA [4].

Some authors suggested that tibial metal augments may not be adequate to fill defects greater than 20 mm, particularly in young patients [5]. Due to this reason and to the lack of versatility of metallic augments, some authors in these cases prefer the use of fresh allograft. The advantages of bone allograft are easy remodeling, ability to fill cavitary or segmental defects, excellent biocompatibility, and potential for ligamentous reattachment. On the contrary, the main concerns regarding bone allograft include late resorption and risk of infectious disease transmission [44].

Considering the poor bone quality and the presence of bone loss, additional (longer) stems are often required in post-traumatic TKA. Brooks et al. demonstrated a reduction of 23–38 % of the axial loads on the tibial component using a 70 mm cemented tibial stem [6]. For this reason, if an augment is necessary, a tibial stem should be used, as well as in cases in which a stronger hinge is necessary because of poor bone or ligamentous quality. The use of stems reduces the axial load to the implant and the bone-cement-implant interface. In the cases where a long diaphyseal bypass is necessary, e.g., in the presence of malunion, a metaphyseal cementation can be performed, in association with long cementless stems [11]. In many cases, there is a lack of congruence between the center of the tibial plateau and the center of the tibial diaphysis: in these cases, most of the authors suggest to use offsetted stems, in order to allow a correct restoration of the tibial surface [3].

12.7   Postoperative Management

The postoperative protocols should not differ from those used in standard TKA. Weight bearing should be calibrated in relation to the primary stability of the implant and can be (rarely) delayed depending on bone grafting and bone reconstruction. If V-Y quadriceps turndown or tibial tubercle osteotomy is used, a more careful

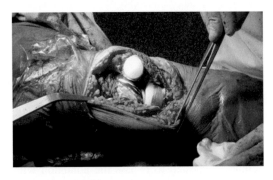

Fig. 12.3 Intraoperative picture showing a tibial wedge

rehabilitation is recommended, to reduce the stresses on the extensor apparatus. In these cases, a hinged brace can be used, allowing passive gentle progressive ROM exercises during non-weight-bearing phases [4].

12.8 Complications

The risk factors for complication in TKA for post-traumatic arthritis include (1) severe stiffness, (2) multiple prior surgeries, (3) prior infection, and (4) poor skin conditions. One of the most serious complications is the avulsion of the patellar tendon; in cases of stiff knee, a more careful exposure, maybe using a tibial tubercle osteotomy, is recommended.

Also skin necrosis is a severe complication and can be correlated with implant exposure and infection. Patients with multiple scars are at high risk of cutaneous necrosis and need to be evaluated by the plastic surgeon preoperatively [27].

There is some concern about the higher risk of peri-prosthetic joint infection in TKA following prior fracture compared to standard TKA. Larson et al. hypothesized that TKAs performed after infected tibial plateau fractures would have a higher complication rate when compared with noninfected tibial plateau fractures. In this case-control study, the authors concluded that previously infected knees had a 4.1-fold increased risk of requiring additional procedures [19]. Recently other authors reported similar results in their case series [24]. In addition, Suzuki et al. evaluated 2022 primary TKA and, using logistic regression analysis, identified having a previous fracture and remnants of internal fixation as a major risk factor for infection [42].

12.9 Results

There are few reports describing the outcomes of TKA in post-traumatic arthritis, with small case series and only short- to medium-term follow-up.

In 1979 Marmor et al. described the results of 18 patients affected by post-traumatic arthritis treated with a modular unicondylar arthroplasty. In 15 cases both the medial and lateral compartments were resurfaced. The authors reported 78 % of satisfactory results 2 years after surgery [26]. Roffi et al. in 1990 described the outcomes of 17 cases of TKA in post-traumatic arthritis, with only 8 successful results. The authors concluded that the results of TKA in these patients may resemble revision rather than primary TKA [35]. However, most authors agree that TKAs after periarticular knee fractures achieve good clinical outcomes, but the procedure can be technically demanding and is associated with a higher failure and complication rate compared to standard TKA [4, 8, 21, 36, 37, 46, 47, 49]. Lizaur-Utrilla et al., in a prospective matched cohort study, evaluated the results of 29 patients affected by post-traumatic arthritis and 58 patients who underwent routine TKA, at 6.7 years of follow-up. The authors concluded that there were no differences in clinical outcomes, but the group affected by post-traumatic arthritis had a significant higher incidence of complications [20]. The results are even less satisfactory in cases of previous malunion or nonunion [32]. There is also a general agreement in affirming that patients affected by isolated intra-articular deformities obtain the better outcomes than more complex cases [38].

Similar results were reported for TKA after prior distal femoral fracture. Papadopoulos et al. reported the results of 47 cemented condylar TKAs in patients affected by previous distal femoral fracture, at an average follow-up of 6.2 years. In three cases, a distal femoral osteotomy in conjunction with longer cemented femoral stem was required because of malunion. The authors reported good clinical outcomes and improved Knee Society pain score and postoperative ROM, but six knee required revision surgery because of arthrofibrosis or aseptic loosening [30].

Considering the problems encountered in patients with prior hardware, such as difficulties in using intramedullary guides, some authors advocated using computer-assisted navigation to perform TKA in post-traumatic arthritis [25].

Table 12.1 shows a summary of the literature on results of TKA after post-traumatic arthritis.

Table 12.1 Summary of the literature regarding TKA in post-traumatic arthritis (ROM=range of motion)

Authors	Year	Number	Diagnosis	Mean follow-up	Outcomes
Marmor [26]	1979	18 knees	Post-traumatic arthritis	2 years	78 % of satisfactory results with modular unicondylar arthroplasty (15 cases of medial and lateral replacement)
Roffi [35]	1990	17 knees	Post-traumatic arthritis	27 months	62 % of patients met the criteria for successful outcome (Hospital for Special Surgery). Five major intraoperative or postoperative complications
Lonner [21]	1999	31 knees	Post-traumatic arthritis	46 months	58 % of good-excellent functional scores and 71 % of good-excellent knee scores. 57 % of complications
Saleh [36]	2001	15 knees	Previous tibial plateau fracture	6.2 years	12 knees scored as good or excellent according to average Hospital for Special Surgery knee score. There was a high rate of infection (3 patients), patellar tendon disruption (2 patients), and postoperative secondary procedures (3 patients required closed manipulation)
Papadopoulos [30]	2002	47 knees	Previous distal femoral fracture	6.2 years	Improved Knee Society pain score and postoperative ROM. Four cases of stiffness treated with Manipulation Under Anesthesia, two aseptic loosening, three deep infections
Weiss [46, 47]	2003	62 knees	Previous tibial plateau fracture	4.7 years	Good results at the knee score. 12 reoperations. 10 % of intraoperative and 26 % of postoperative complication rates
Wu [49]	2005	15 knees	Post-traumatic arthritis	35 months	Good results in terms of the knee score. The mean ROM was 94° at the last follow-up. 4 postoperative stiff knees requiring manipulation under anesthesia
Larson [19]	2009	19 knee	Previous infected tibial plateau fracture	6.4 years	53 % of complications and 26 % of recurrent infection
Civinini [8]	2009	29 knees	Post-traumatic arthritis	92 months	8 % of implant failure
Parratte [32]	2011	74 knees	Post-traumatic arthritis	4 years	Good clinical outcomes. 26 % of complications, most of all with severe consequence on functional outcomes (three extensor system avulsions, four infections, five cases of stiffness, and one of instability)
Shearer [38]	2013	47 knees	Post-traumatic arthritis	52 months	Significant improvement in Knee Society pain score. Better results in patients affected by isolated articular deformities. Soft tissue defects requiring flap coverage were associated with worsening of the pain score ($p=0.027$)

Authors	Year	Number	Diagnosis	Mean follow-up	Outcomes
Lunebourg [24]	2014	33 knees	Post-traumatic arthritis	11 years	Greater improvement in the control group of elective TKAs ($p < 0.001$), with associated greater improvement in ROM ($p = 0.001$). The survival rate of TKA at 10 years was better in the elective TKAs group (99 %, CI: 98–100 vs. 79 %, CI: 69–89; $p < 0.001$)
Benazzo [4]	2014	44 knees	Post-traumatic arthritis	6 years	22 posterior-stabilized (PS) implants, 22 condylar constrained (CCK) implants. Good functional outcomes at the final follow-up. No differences between PS and CCK
Manzotti [25]	2014	16 knees	Post-traumatic after distal femoral fracture and retained hardware	Not reported	Group I: post-traumatic arthritis with navigated TKA. Group II: arthritis with navigated TKA (matched paired). No significant differences in surgical time, hospital staying, or intraoperative and postoperative complications between the two study groups
Lizaur-Utrilla [20]	2015	29 knee (matched with 58 standard TKA)	Post-traumatic arthritis	6.7 years	Comparable clinical results in the two groups. In post-traumatic arthritis higher incidence of minor complications
Scott [37]	2015	31 knees	Post-traumatic arthritis	>60 months	Higher complication rates compared to a match-paired group of standard TKA (13 % vs. 1 %)

Conclusion

The incidence of post-traumatic arthritis is reported in literature ranging between 20 % at 5 years and 50 % at 15 years after a proximal tibial fracture. TKA after proximal tibia or distal femoral fracture is a more demanding procedure compared to standard TKA. When approaching a knee replacement in a patient with previous surgery, the strategy should be accurately planned because of different problems: hardware presence, multiple surgical scars, stiffness, bony defects, malalignment, instability, malunion, and previous infections. A comprehensive preoperative planning is mandatory in these patients, in order to choose the correct implant and to better evaluate bone loss. There are few reports in the literature regarding TKA in posttraumatic arthritis, but most of those papers conclude that the outcomes are more similar to revision than to primary TKA. In addition, due to the previous surgery, more difficult exposure, and surgical technique, the incidence of complications after TKA in post-traumatic arthritis is higher than standard TKA.

References

1. Amendola A, Bonasia DE (2010) Results of high tibial osteotomy: review of the literature. Int Orthop 34(2):155–160. doi:10.1007/s00264-009-0889-8
2. Anderson SP, Matthews LS, Kaufer H (1990) Treatment of juxtaarticular nonunion fractures at the knee with long-stem total knee arthroplasty. Clin Orthop Relat Res 260:104–109
3. Bedi A, Haidukewych GJ (2009) Management of the posttraumatic arthritic knee. J Am Acad Orthop Surg 17(2):88–101
4. Benazzo F, Rossi SM, Ghiara M, Zanardi A, Perticarini L, Combi A (2014) Total knee replacement in acute and chronic traumatic events. Injury 45(Suppl 6):S98–S104. doi:10.1016/j.injury.2014.10.031
5. Brand MG, Daley RJ, Ewald FC, Scott RD (1989) Tibial tray augmentation with modular metal wedges for tibial bone stock deficiency. Clin Orthop Relat Res 248:71–79
6. Brooks PJ, Walker PS, Scott RD (1984) Tibial component fixation in deficient tibial bone stock. Clin Orthop Relat Res 184:302–308
7. Buechel FF (2002) Knee arthroplasty in post-traumatic arthritis. J Arthroplasty 17(4 Suppl 1):63–68
8. Civinini R, Carulli C, Matassi F, Villano M, Innocenti M (2009) Total knee arthroplasty after complex tibial plateau fractures. La Chirurgia degli organi di movimento 93(3):143–147. doi:10.1007/s12306-009-0033-3
9. Court-Brown CM, Bugler KE, Clement ND, Duckworth AD, McQueen MM (2012) The epidemiology of open fractures in adults. A 15-year review. Injury 43(6):891–897. doi:10.1016/j.injury.2011.12.007
10. Della Valle CJ, Berger RA, Rosenberg AG (2006) Surgical exposures in revision total knee arthroplasty. Clin Orthop Relat Res 446:59–68. doi:10.1097/01.blo.0000214434.64774.d5
11. Dennis DA (2002) The structural allograft composite in revision total knee arthroplasty. J Arthroplasty 17(4 Suppl 1):90–93
12. Dettoni F, Bonasia DE, Castoldi F, Bruzzone M, Blonna D, Rossi R (2010) High tibial osteotomy versus unicompartmental knee arthroplasty for medial compartment arthrosis of the knee: a review of the literature. Iowa Orthop J 30:131–140
13. Haidukewych GJ, Hanssen A, Jones RD (2011) Metaphyseal fixation in revision total knee arthroplasty: indications and techniques. J Am Acad Orthop Surg 19(6):311–318
14. Honkonen SE (1995) Degenerative arthritis after tibial plateau fractures. J Orthop Trauma 9(4):273–277
15. Johnson DP (1993) Infection after knee arthroplasty. Clinical studies of skin hypoxia and wound healing. Acta Orthop Scand Suppl 252:1–48
16. Kettelkamp DB, Hillberry BM, Murrish DE, Heck DA (1988) Degenerative arthritis of the knee secondary to fracture malunion. Clin Orthop Relat Res 234:159–169
17. Kotani A, Yonekura A, Bourne RB (2005) Factors influencing range of motion after contemporary total knee arthroplasty. J Arthroplasty 20(7):850–856. doi:10.1016/j.arth.2004.12.051
18. Kress KJ, Scuderi GR, Windsor RE, Insall JN (1993) Treatment of nonunions about the knee utilizing custom total knee arthroplasty with press-fit intramedullary stems. J Arthroplasty 8(1):49–55
19. Larson AN, Hanssen AD, Cass JR (2009) Does prior infection alter the outcome of TKA after tibial plateau fracture? Clin Orthop Relat Res 467(7):1793–1799. doi:10.1007/s11999-008-0615-7
20. Lizaur-Utrilla A, Collados-Maestre I, Miralles-Munoz FA, Lopez-Prats FA (2015) Total knee arthroplasty for osteoarthritis secondary to fracture of the Tibial Plateau. A Prospective Matched Cohort Study. J Arthroplasty 30(8):1328–1332. doi:10.1016/j.arth.2015.02.032
21. Lonner JH, Pedlow FX, Siliski JM (1999) Total knee arthroplasty for post-traumatic arthrosis. J Arthroplasty 14(8):969–975
22. Lonner JH, Siliski JM, Jupiter JB, Lhowe DW (1999) Posttraumatic nonunion of the proximal tibial metaphysis. Am J Orthop 28(9):523–528
23. Lonner JH, Siliski JM, Lotke PA (2000) Simultaneous femoral osteotomy and total knee arthroplasty for treatment of osteoarthritis associated with severe extra-articular deformity. J Bone Joint Surg Am 82(3):342–348

24. Lunebourg A, Parratte S, Gay A, Ollivier M, Garcia-Parra K, Argenson JN (2015) Lower function, quality of life, and survival rate after total knee arthroplasty for posttraumatic arthritis than for primary arthritis. Acta Orthop 86(2):189–194. doi:10.3109/17453674.2014.979723

25. Manzotti A, Pullen C, Cerveri P, Chemello C, Confalonieri N (2014) Post traumatic knee arthritis: navigated total knee replacement without hardware removal. Knee 21(1):290–294. doi:10.1016/j.knee.2012.06.008

26. Marmor L (1979) The Marmot modular knee in traumatic arthritis. Orthop Rev 8:35

27. Massin P, Bonnin M, Paratte S, Vargas R, Piriou P, Deschamps G, French Hip Knee S (2011) Total knee replacement in post-traumatic arthritic knees with limitation of flexion. Orthop Traumatol Surg Res 97(1):28–33. doi:10.1016/j.otsr.2010.06.016

28. Massin P, Lautridou C, Cappelli M, Petit A, Odri G, Ducellier F, Sabatier C, Hulet C, Canciani JP, Letenneur J, Burdin P, Societe d'Orthopedie de lO (2009) Total knee arthroplasty with limitations of flexion. Orthop Traumatol Surg Res 95(4 Suppl 1): S1–S6. doi:10.1016/j.otsr.2009.04.002

29. Menderes A, Demirdover C, Yilmaz M, Vayvada H, Barutcu A (2002) Reconstruction of soft tissue defects following total knee arthroplasty. Knee 9(3):215–219

30. Papadopoulos EC, Parvizi J, Lai CH, Lewallen DG (2002) Total knee arthroplasty following prior distal femoral fracture. Knee 9(4):267–274

31. Papagelopoulos PJ, Partsinevelos AA, Themistocleous GS, Mavrogenis AF, Korres DS, Soucacos PN (2006) Complications after tibia plateau fracture surgery. Injury 37(6):475–484. doi:10.1016/j.injury.2005.06.035

32. Parratte S, Boyer P, Piriou P, Argenson JN, Deschamps G, Massin P, SFHG (2011) Total knee replacement following intra-articular malunion. Orthop Traumatol Surg Res 97(6 Suppl):S118–S123. doi:10.1016/j.otsr.2011.07.001

33. Radnay CS, Scuderi GR (2006) Management of bone loss: augments, cones, offset stems. Clin Orthop Relat Res 446:83–92. doi:10.1097/01.blo.0000214437.57151.41

34. Rasmussen PS (1972) Tibial condylar fractures as a cause of degenerative arthritis. Acta Orthop Scand 43(6):566–575

35. Roffi RP, Merritt PO (1990) Total knee replacement after fractures about the knee. Orthop Rev 19(7):614–620

36. Saleh KJ, Sherman P, Katkin P, Windsor R, Haas S, Laskin R, Sculco T (2001) Total knee arthroplasty after open reduction and internal fixation of fractures of the tibial plateau: a minimum five-year follow-up study. J Bone Joint Surg Am 83-A(8):1144–1148

37. Scott CE, Davidson E, MacDonald DJ, White TO, Keating JF (2015) Total knee arthroplasty following tibial plateau fracture: a matched cohort study. Bone Joint J 97-B(4):532–538. doi:10.1302/0301-620X.97B4.34789

38. Shearer DW, Chow V, Bozic KJ, Liu J, Ries MD (2013) The predictors of outcome in total knee arthroplasty for post-traumatic arthritis. Knee 20(6):432–436. doi:10.1016/j.knee.2012.12.010

39. Siliski JM, Mahring M, Hofer HP (1989) Supracondylar-intercondylar fractures of the femur. Treatment by internal fixation. J Bone Joint Surg Am 71(1):95–104

40. Springer BD, Hanssen AD, Sim FH, Lewallen DG (2001) The kinematic rotating hinge prosthesis for complex knee arthroplasty. Clin Orthop Relat Res 392:283–291

41. Stahl JP, Alt V, Kraus R, Hoerbelt R, Itoman M, Schnettler R (2006) Derotation of post-traumatic femoral deformities by closed intramedullary sawing. Injury 37(2):145–151. doi:10.1016/j.injury.2005.06.042

42. Suzuki G, Saito S, Ishii T, Motojima S, Tokuhashi Y, Ryu J (2011) Previous fracture surgery is a major risk factor of infection after total knee arthroplasty. Knee Surg Sports Traumatol Arthrosc (Official Journal of the ESSKA) 19(12):2040–2044. doi:10.1007/s00167-011-1525-x

43. Tarabichi S, Tarabichi Y (2010) Can an anterior quadriceps release improve range of motion in the stiff arthritic knee? J Arthroplasty 25(4):571–575. doi:10.1016/j.arth.2009.04.015

44. Tigani D, Dallari D, Coppola C, Ben Ayad R, Sabbioni G, Fosco M (2011) Total knee arthroplasty for post-traumatic proximal tibial bone defect: three cases report. Open Orthop J 5:143–150. doi:10.2174/1874325001105010143

45. Wasserstein D, Henry P, Paterson JM, Kreder HJ, Jenkinson R (2014) Risk of total knee arthroplasty after operatively treated tibial plateau fracture: a matched-population-based cohort study. J Bone Joint Surg Am 96(2):144–150. doi:10.2106/JBJS.L.01691

46. Weiss NG, Parvizi J, Hanssen AD, Trousdale RT, Lewallen DG (2003) Total knee arthroplasty in post-traumatic arthrosis of the knee. J Arthroplasty 18(3 Suppl 1):23–26. doi:10.1054/arth.2003.50068

47. Weiss NG, Parvizi J, Trousdale RT, Bryce RD, Lewallen DG (2003) Total knee arthroplasty in patients with a prior fracture of the tibial plateau. J Bone Joint Surg Am 85-A(2):218–221

48. Windsor RE, Insall JN, Vince KG (1988) Technical considerations of total knee arthroplasty after proximal tibial osteotomy. J Bone Joint Surg Am 70(4):547–555

49. Wu LD, Xiong Y, Yan SG, Yang QS (2005) Total knee replacement for posttraumatic degenerative arthritis of the knee. Chin J Traumatol (Zhonghua chuang shang za zhi/Chinese Medical Association) 8(4):195–199

50. Yoshino N, Takai S, Watanabe Y, Nakamura S, Kubo T (2004) Total knee arthroplasty with long stem for treatment of nonunion after high tibial osteotomy. J Arthroplasty 19(4):528–531

Printed in the United States
By Bookmasters